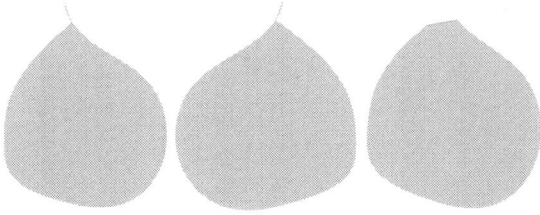

A VERY BEGINNER'S GUIDE TO

Homeopathy

AND FAMILY HEALTH

REBECCA BERMEISTER DIP HOM

In loving dedication
to my darling mother Leah,
who taught her children the sacred nature
of all living creatures.

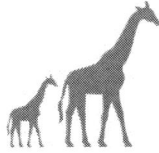

With deepest gratitude to my teacher George Vithoulkas
and the International Academy of Classical Homeopathy,
and to my dear friend Michelle Ofstun
for her sharp editorial eye and gracious time.

As a young mother I was lucky to have been introduced to Homeopathy when a friend sent me to a wonderful homeopath named Leslie Meredith, who became our family practitioner for many years. Later, I met Tamara Lowe who treated our family and to whom I am ever grateful for her insights and support which ultimately led me to study and qualify as a practitioner, with the encouragement of my darling uncle Roy.

Through my daily interactions with patients, I came to realize the need for a very simple introduction to the correct principles of Classical Homeopathy. I remember when I first stumbled upon Homeopathy, I was so intrigued that I just wanted to read everything I could, and I sense this excitement in many of the young parents I meet today. But homeopathy is complicated and easily misunderstood.

While Phyllis Speight's book, *Homeopathy: A Home Prescriber,* was never far from reach, and Tricia Allan's, *Your Healthy Child with Homeopathy* guided me well, it was Vithoulkas's *The Science of Homeopathy*, which really grabbed my attention, grounding the theories of Homeopathy in science. I never imagined then that I would have the opportunity to learn with the esteemed professor and master homeopath himself. Years later I graduated from his school, the International Academy of Classical Homeopathy, and have been a devoted student ever since.

While my intention was to write a simple guide, in all honesty, after studying with Vithoulkas, I came to understand that Homeopathy is not simple. Correct homeopathy should be considered a specialized addition to medicine. Still parents should be encouraged to treat their families with low dose homeopathic remedies for mild acute illnesses and the myriad of mishaps which children encounter in daily family life. Understanding the principles well will allow you to do so with confidence.

Chapters

1. Food, Nutrition and Family health
   - Nutrients & Cell Health
   - Shopping for Change
   - New Moms & Post Natal Care
2. Homeopathy- Nature's Medicine
   - The Law of Similars
   - Understanding the Aggravation
   - Proving the Remedy
   - The Law of Cure
3. Treatments
   - Constitutional Treatment
   - Chronic Treatment
   - Acute Treatment- Physical, Emotional, Mental
   - Preventative Treatment
4. Finding the Remedy- S.I.C.K.
   - Putting the Pieces Together
   - Sensation, Influences, Causes, Keynotes
   - Differentiating Remedies
5. A Deeper Understanding
   - Layers
   - Symptoms
   - Direction of Cure
   - Levels of Health
   - Suppression of Symptoms
   - Hereditary (miasmic) Predispositions
   - Response to the Remedy
   - The Follow Up
6. Healing Takes Time
   - Tuning into the Body
   - Potencies and Dosing
7. Remedies for Home Treatment- Materia Medica
8. Natural Immunity
   - Unpacking Vaccines
9. Recipes- My Cauldron
   - Medicine Pantry
   - Vaccine Education Resources, Books and References

CHAPTER 1

Food, Nutrition & Family health

Before you heal someone, ask him first if he is willing to
give up the things which make him sick.

Hypocrites

Heavily pregnant with the first of my five children, I hauled myself up the carpeted stairs of the Victorian building in one of Sydney's more bohemian inner-city suburbs and entered the demonstration kitchen which sat above the iconic street-front macrobiotic restaurant, IKU. A friend had recommended the cooking class which was the perfect introduction for me. Even though I grew up in a home where the pantry was full and the kitchen warm, I never showed much interest in food until I fell pregnant- then all I wanted to do was eat.

Here, cooking was taught as a meditation, grounded in the natural world of the elements and aligned with the teachings of traditional Japanese customs and the principles of Tao- the harmony of opposites. Meat and chicken are yang, sugar and fruits are yin. Slow-cooked root vegetables such as sweet potato and pumpkin are grounding, which is more yang, while sweet fruits supply fast yin energy.

We came to understand how cooked foods are easier to digest while raw foods use up digestive heat (fire) to break them down. This is fine in summer if you're young with a strong digestive system, but require too much energy in the cooler months, especially if you are elderly, frail or recovering from illness or childbirth- then, you should favor soups, stews and slow baked warming vegetables. Food is generally selected by season and climate, and for the individual- taking into account their disposition, occupation and state of health.

Encouraged to sit quietly and eat with awareness, in a calm environment, chewing each mouth-full well to aid in the mechanical breakdown of our food making it easier to digest, we explored the relationship between food and the body – 'you are what you eat', being a founding truth. Traditional Japanese cooking which rests on macrobiotic principles, brings this awareness to food selection and preparation- from the ground to the table.

Traditional Japanese chefs are masters, the preparation of food is a meditation which you sense and taste with each delicious mouthful.

We learned how to cut vegetables so that each slice contains both yin and yang, to chew our rice 100 times, and, most importantly, that a chocolate cake made by grandma with love, can nourish you more than the healthiest meal.

We explored how nature gives us clues about plant's curative abilities. Cut a carrot into rounds and see the human eye- carrots provide beta-Carotene, which is converted to vitamin A, needed for good eye health. Walnuts resemble the brain and are high in omega 3 fatty acids which boost memory. Tomatoes have four rich, red chambers, and resemble the human heart. They are high in antioxidants, specifically anthocyanin which reduce risk factors for heart disease and help lower blood pressure and cholesterol. This is called the Doctrine of Signatures, and it has been used in folk medicine since man first roamed the planet. It is also a tenet of Homeopathy- like cures like.

Ayurveda is much the same, in principle. Certain foods cool us down, while others warm us up. Some of us are more earthy, sluggish, damp and sweet, others run hot with a fast metabolism and are industrious and easily stressed. Ayurveda recommends specific foods, herbs, spices and combinations which suit the individual's metabolism and temperament. The wisdom of the ancient Indian healing system is grounded in thousands of years of tradition and a thorough understanding of the elements, and the knowledge that the individual's state of health needs to be evaluated in the context of their temperament, nature, environment and physiology. Nothing exists as a separate entity; everything is connected. Mind, body, spirit, soul, energy, breath, nature, food.

Likewise, Traditional Chinese Medicine is founded on the ancient understanding of the embodiment of the elements; wood, water, fire, earth and air. These elements are expressed in the systems and organs of the physical body, and the flow of energy between them directs physicians to understand where imbalance and disharmony take place. The tools of acupuncture, tongue and pulse diagnosis, shiatsu, and Chinese herbs, allow physicians to redirect that flow, encouraging movement where there is stagnation and bringing balance and harmony. The elements, which animate the flow of energy between the organs and systems have emotional, mental and spiritual expressions which are integrated into the healing process. There is little separation between the grief of a broken heart and the lung infection which follows; bring one into order and the other will naturally follow, not via suppression, but via flow of the vital life force, the Chi.

In homeopathy too, human systems are inter-connected, and we examine each with equal interest. The cognitive/mental, emotional and physical health of the individual provides essential information and guides us towards the selection of the correct remedy and sequence of remedies required to progress the organism towards health on all levels.

In his book, *Levels of Health,* master homeopath George Vithoulkas defines health as follows:

> *Freedom from pain and the attainment of a state of well-being in the physical body, freedom from passion and the attainment of a state of calm in the emotional body, and freedom from selfishness and the attainment of unification with truth in the mental body.*
>
> *The measure of health, is the degree to which a person is free to be creative and productive (as opposed to destructive), promoting the interests of good for oneself and for others[1].*

For a healing method to be complete it must integrate all the parts of the whole. Only modern medicine (and her cohort, modern science), separates us into organs and systems; as if the skin has nothing to do with the digestive system, as if the digestive system has nothing to do with the immune system, as if the immune system has nothing to do with the emotional state. We are complex, multi-lingual beings, we speak many languages: the language of touch, the language of intimacy, the language of social response. The body speaks her own language, as does the soul. All systems feed into one another effecting our sense of health and wellbeing. Nothing exists on its own.

---

[1] Levels of Health, 2nd volume 3rd revised edition, George Vithoulkas. (My bracketed addition for clarification)

NUTRIENTS & CELL HEALTH

I begin our journey with food because it is essential to understand the importance quality nutrients play in our health. We tend to not think too much about the relationship between food and the body, but the food we eat is literally our fuel. We are organisms living in nature, our energy comes directly from the water we drink, the oxygen we breath, the sun in which we bathe, the earth on which we walk, the company we keep and the food we eat, not just physically but energetically as well.

> *You may consider yourself an individual, but as a cell biologist, I can tell you that you are in truth a cooperative community of approximately fifty trillion single celled citizens. Almost all of the cells that make your body are amoeba like individual organisms that have evolved a cooperative strategy for their natural survival.*
>
> *Bruce H Lipton, PhD.*

For those new to biology a quick and simple introduction. Cells make up all the tissues in the body. Tissues line all the walls of all our organs and vessels, connecting, protecting and insulating them. Cells make up our muscles, nerves, blood, cartilage and bones. They make up the brain, the heart, the lungs, the liver, the gall bladder, the pancreas, the stomach, the reproductive and urinary organs. Organs work together in systems; the nervous system, the cardiovascular system, the endocrine system, the digestive system, the lymphatic system, the reproductive system, the genitourinary system, the muscular system. Systems make up the organism, commonly known as you. You are almost entirely made from cells.

Cells are the building blocks of the body. They fight disease, transport oxygen, store nutrients, make proteins, they grow, they reproduce, they fight, they react. But most importantly, they transform nutrients into energy. We use this energy for everything we do. From moving our eyeball across a line of text, to picking up our miserable toddler in the middle of the night for a cuddle. We also use this energy for all the things we do unconsciously- the functions of autonomic nervous system. These include the hormonal, cardiovascular, digestive and lung functions to name a few. Cellular energy powers everything we do. Cells do all of their jobs using the fuel we provide them by the foods we eat and the oxygen we breath.

The food is broken down by mechanical (chewing) and chemical (digestion) processes, and nutrients are slowly absorbed through the semi porous intestinal walls into the blood. Small molecules including glucose (from the food we eat), pass into the intercellular fluid and through the semi-permeable cell membrane into the cell itself where it is further broken down and transformed to produce energy. The cells power the whole organism and the nutrients power the cells. We are literally what we eat.

In her wonderful book *Nourishing Traditions,* Sally Fallon writes about the health benefits of traditional food preparation, storage, and cooking methods. Cultures who have maintained their traditional food customs, are no doubt healthier than those of us who have sacrificed ours in exchange for modern conveniences such as microwaves and pre-cooked and packaged foods.

Not that long ago, fresh vegetables were preserved with salts, creating lactic acid via the natural fermentation process providing important nutrients and probiotics which aid in digestion. Milk when fermented converts the lactose and casein protein many of us have trouble with, into lactic acid (which helps break down lactose). Buttermilks, soured milks, yogurts, and kefir are rich in vitamins B and C, which increase with fermentation. Before the industrialization of food, all bread was sour dough made from a living starter culture of local yeast. (See recipe for making your own easy starter culture and fermented vegetables in chapter 8).

Food was never intended for mass production and industrialization. Commercial foods need to be preserved to ensure a long shelf life and to withstand transportation and storage. Today, store bought food is mostly dead food, void of micro-nutrients, living cultures, energy and life-force. Modern farming methods have stripped our soil of so much of her goodness, produce is sprayed with known carcinogenic pesticides and our foods are more poison than they are good. The food industry, along with the advertising industry, has intentionally distanced us from our food traditions, our connection to the healing earth and her natural medicinal gifts.

With the industrialization of the modern kitchen and with all the promises of saved time and convenience, our children do not know how to make bread, or pickle olives. Exchanging tradition for convenience in our homes and kitchens is one of the greatest tragedies of our time. We have traded our health and the health of our families for false promises. But we can make changes starting with what we bring into our kitchens and our homes.

SHOPPING FOR CHANGE

While fathers by their very nature, are protectors and providers, mothers are nurturers and healers. We are called on to be medicine women to our families, and our medicine comes primarily from our gardens and our kitchens. Your kitchen is your storehouse of nutrients, the place where food is transformed into nourishing meals. Your family will mostly eat what you grow, what you bring into your home and what you cook, so chose carefully what you load into your shopping cart. Fresh, local and seasonal is best.

Start in the fruit and vegetable section of your supermarket and load up your trolly with fresh, local and preferably organic produce. Buy enough fresh tomatoes to make your own sauces for home-made pizza and pasta, and enough free-range eggs to make your own mayonnaise. Buy plenty of fresh herbs, so you can turn a simple pot of basmati rice into a Persian delight, and enough seeds, nuts and dried fruit so you can nibble on healthy snacks and teach your children to do the same.

Then head towards the health isles and fill up with raw honey, good oils (see below), additive free sauces, miso paste, naturally brewed or fermented soy sauce, condiments, a variety of grains, legumes, pasta, noodles and spices. We have been led to believe that all fat, salt and sugar are bad, but we need to differentiate between good and bad fats, salts and sugars.

Good fats include grass fed butters, olive oil, avocado and coconut oils as well as cold pressed vegetable oils. If you deep fry from time to time, use a cold pressed vegetable oil with a high smoke point such as grape seed (not to be confused with Rapeseed/Canola which is highly toxic), or rice-bran oil. If you refrigerate a pot of chicken soup overnight, in the morning you can scrape off the chicken fat and use it as a spread. Duck and goose fats are stable fats and can be used for frying. Fish fats are an excellent source of omega three.

Good salts are those which have not been stripped of their minerals through processing; watch out for free-flowing agents and added iodine, these are unnecessary and toxic additions to table salt. Look for pink Himalayan salts, kosher, raw cooking salts, raw sea salts-damp and grey in color in their natural form, they are rich in mineral content. Salts are great to add to a warm bath. High in magnesium, they will settle a hyperactive child after a day in a highly chlorinated pool, and they will calm the nerves of an exhausted parent who has pushed themselves too far.

Epsom salt (not for eating) is excellent to add to a bath at the end of a long day when you need to relax tired muscles. In children with behavioral challenges, a cup of Epsom salt added to a bath every day will help settle an overstimulated nervous system. It will help your child sleep and settle better. Many children on the spectrum have been found to be low in Sulphate. The Sulphur in Epsom Salt is in the correct form (sulphate) so it is easily absorbed and utilized[2] in the natural detoxification of phenols, which are found in fruit and vegetables, preservatives, medicines and household cleaning products. If your child is on the spectrum, it's a good idea to look at foods high in phenols and reduce them while you build up their sulphates and their healthy gut bacteria.

Good sugars include: maple syrup, agave, stevia and raw honeys, malt syrups, rice syrups and some forms of natural molasses. Sweet cravings can be satisfied by increasing your intake of sweet vegetables such as pumpkin, beets, sweet potato, corn, and fruits such as dates, sultanas, dried fruits etc.

Grains, beans and legumes MUST be soaked well before being cooked. Phytates in legumes interfere with the absorption of nutrients and are reduced with pre-soaking. Almost all grains, seeds and nuts can be sprouted (at home, with a simple glass jar and some water), and

---

[2] https://www.mgwater.com/transdermal.shtml - Dr Rosemary Waring

should be a welcome addition to family meals and snacks. Sprouts make a simple salad special and add much needed vitamins and enzymes.

Almost everything can be made at home and the internet is full of easy recipes to follow, but if you don't have time, read ingredient contents well and chose products whose ingredients list you understand. For example, choose applesauce made from: apples, sea-salt, water and ascorbic acid (vitamin C) instead of ones to which preservatives, color, flavor and sugar have been added. If a product has more than five or six ingredients, and a list of numbers and names that read like a chemistry class, it is probably best left on the shelf.

Shop together with your partner and share articles and information on nutrition, so that once the children arrive, food doesn't become a source of tension between you. You can buy delicious and healthy treats and snacks from health food markets. Good quality dark chocolate has a place in everyone's pantry, as does a big bag of sea salt or chili-lime potato or vegetable chips. You can be healthy and enjoy your food, you just have to source good replacements for commercial rubbish, which I suggest you flush straight down the toilet, and avoid the middleman!

Utensils are important too. Think about the quality of your pots, pans and cooking equipment. Pots and pans should be made from natural materials- stainless steel and cast iron. Non-stick aluminum cookware leaches and should not be used. Teflon is toxic. Choose wooden or bamboo utensils and chopping boards, glass and ceramic bowls and storage containers, and never put hot foods into plastic. Avoid cooking in aluminum foil. Aluminum has been found in the brains of those suffering from Alzheimer's and Autism[3]. Choose paper and cotton cloth over plastic and foil wherever possible. And consider the earth on which we roam. She too has to eat the garbage we throw into her. Chose bamboo or plant-based and recycle-able one-time use cutlery if you need to use it, and bring your own coffee mug where possible.

---

[3] Professor Chris Exley - Aluminium in Human Brain Tissue
https://www.hippocraticpost.com/pharmacy-drugs/aluminium-in-human-brain-tissue

NEW MOMS AND POST NATAL CARE

Most expectant moms have already started to eat well during or prior to falling pregnant, so you probably already know what you like. Before the birth of your baby, make a list of meals you would like to receive and share it with family and friends you expect might visit after the birth. Limit visits to twenty minutes and ask anyone who comes to bring a meal. If visitors ask if they can help, train your partner and yourself to say YES. Find small chores you need done and give yourself permission to accept help. Close family and friends will be more than happy to fold a load of washing, wash the dishes in the sink, or sweep the floor. These seemingly simple tasks are not your business when you have a new baby to care for and are recovering from birth. And, you set a healthy precedent, so they will feel comfortable asking for help when they need it.

Meals should be nourishing and warming; slow cooked soups and broths, slow roasted root vegetables, udon noodles, miso soup, organic chicken and fish, basmati rice-simple, nourishing and easy to digest. Avoid strong spices unless you have grown up with them. Avoid the cabbage and broccoli families (cruciferous vegetables), deep fried foods and stay away from all dairy products for the first six weeks if you are breastfeeding your baby. Chocolate and coffee should also be avoided while breast-feeding. Make sure to drink plenty of clear fluids. That means every time you get up to pee, come back with a glass of water or herb tea. Diluted apple juice is gentle on the stomach and provides the right pH balance- 1:7 apple juice: water. Don't worry too much about the sugar, most new moms can do with a little extra glucose energy, but again, if you drink a whole bottle of apple juice every day, that's too much. One or two glasses is not going to do any harm.

I also advise new moms not to think about losing weight until they have weaned their babies. You are a feeding machine, surrender and enjoy. If you are feeding well, the weight will come off naturally over the course of your feeding years. If not, you can deal with it later. A nursing mom should not be thinking about losing weight, she should be thinking about supplying quality nutrients to herself and to her child.

In traditional Chinese homes, the women folk take care of the new mother whose job is to rest, recover, replenish and feed her infant. Hot meals are delivered, and she does not participate in household chores for the first few months, nor does she wash her hair or bathe in cold water. Post-natal depression is less common, because the impact of birthing and feeding a newborn is respected. In the west we are so quick to get back on our feet, to be social and engage with the world, returning to work and household chores too quickly. If we don't respect the primal power of birth, we deplete our energy and suffer later. We need to nurture ourselves to recover well, and often this takes a village. The feminist movement has done nothing in our favor by encouraging us back into the workforce too soon after birthing our young.

◖◖◖

CHAPTER 2

Homeopathy ~ Nature's medicine

By similar things, a disease is produced, and through the application
of the like, (the disease) is cured.

Hippocrates

During the early 1800s, the founding father of Homeopathy, Dr Samuel Hahnemann, began experimenting with dilutions of the common medicines of the day, in an attempt to reduce their harsh side effects. Hahnemann and his colleagues found that very well-diluted and potentized (succussed) medicines retained something of their original imprint and were equally if not more effective in treating their patients, and they left no lasting damaging side effects. Patients were able to recover from their illness without having to also recover from the damage done by the drugs they were given.

Hahnemann's stated intention, which can be found in his Organon of Medicine, is *to ensure the rapid, gentle and permanent restoration of health by the complete removal of the disease, in the shortest, most reliable and most harmless way*; and so, homeopathy was born.

Today, the Homeopathic Materia Medica (list of remedies), is made up of hundreds of remedies from the mineral, plant and animal kingdoms, as well as sarcodes (secretions) and nosodes (pathogens). Homeopathic pharmacists dilute and succuss these raw materials until the particles are activated and refined in a way that allows them to induce rapid, gentle and lasting change. Since nothing of the original toxic substance remains, cure takes place without (lasting) negative side effect. So, when you do a search for the remedy Syphilinum (from syphilis) or Lachesis (from snake venom), you can rest assured that the remedy you have been prescribed contains nothing but an imprint of its original toxic substance.

How does this differ from modern pharmaceutical-based medicine? Pharmaceutical medicines are chemicals which trick the body into suppressing its own natural chemical reaction. For example, Protein Pump Inhibitors (PPI's) suppress the production of stomach acid, which can cause reflux, GERD, and stomach ulcers. Beta blockers, ACE Inhibitors and calcium channel blockers are common blood pressure medications. You can see by their names, that they are suppressive in nature. Paracetamol (Acetaminophen) also called Tylenol, Panadol and Calpol, inhibits the synthesis of prostaglandin in the central nervous system. And Ibuprofen, (NSAID's- non-steroid anti-inflammatory), branded as Advil, Motrin and Pedia-Care, reduce hormones that cause inflammation.

Antibiotics destroy good and bad bacteria. When the bacteria are life-threatening, antibiotics can be a godsend, but for the last forty years, they have been misused, creating generations of patients with abysmal gut bacteria and an array of associated behavioral and mental health issues[4], not to mention digestive complaints. Paracetamol has also been associated with a lack of empathy in those who use it. It seems not only to kill our own pain, but our ability to empathize with the pain of others[5].

Steroids (corticosteroids) are anti-inflammatory and immunosuppressive. They work by inactivating a pathway inside the cells (called the nuclear factor KapaB pathway), which suppresses the production of inflammatory cells. Steroids are used to treat allergies, bronchial issues, asthma, eczema and inflammatory bone, joint and tissue diseases such as rheumatoid arthritis. The list of side effects of each of these medications is longer than my arm. It has been pointed out that the term 'side effects' is incorrect. That these *effects* of the drugs we take and give to our children so easily, should be considered as important as the immediate relief they provide. What is the price we pay for that immediate relief?

Pain, inflammation and infection are not your enemy, they are your alarm. But if you shut down your alarm every time it rings, eventually you will wear down the mechanism and it will stop alerting you to the fact that something is wrong. The immune system creates pain and inflammation to alert the immune system to produce and activate killer cells to fight the invading pathogens. The pain and discomfort also inform us to stop, take note, rest, attune, clean, circulate, slow down, massage, nourish, hydrate. Suppressive chemicals are a snooze

---

[4] The Gut Microbiome and Mental Health: Implications for Anxiety- and Trauma-Related Disorders. Pubmed.
Stefanie Malan-Muller 1 , Mireia Valles-Colomer 2   3 , Jeroen Raes 2   3 , Christopher A Lowry 4 5 6 7 8 , Soraya Seedat 1 ,
Sian M J Hemmings 1

[5] https://academic.oup.com/scan/article/11/9/1345/2224135 - From Painkiller to Empathy Killer: acetaminophen (paracetamol) reduces empathy for pain.

button, which allow us to continue in a state of slumber. If we use them too often, we risk oversleeping, missing the train and creating a health crisis further down the track.

We have grown up with these common medications without respecting them. There is a time and a place for pharmaceutical medications; emergency care, surgery, end of life palliation, replacement of essential hormones like insulin and thyroid hormones, HIV medications, cancer treatments, serious organ disease treatments and essential lifesaving and life prolonging medications- miraculous discoveries worthy of great respect.

Homeopathy does not oppose modern medicine, but rather it is a refined and advanced arm of modern medicine. It brings something infinitely more advanced and holistic to the healing process, supporting medicine by providing a very refined mechanism which is highly effective and completely safe without adding any additional, unnecessary toxic load. It is the future of intelligent medicine.

The Law of Similars - like cures like

The patient's symptoms are a compass for the homeopath to find the correct remedy. Vithoulkas

When taken by healthy volunteers, a remedy is proven, meaning it produces a set of symptoms. For example, when taken by a healthy volunteer, the highly toxic plant Belladonna, (in a diluted and potentized form) will produce a sudden high fever, red flushed cheeks and dilated pupils, while Mercurius (mercury) will produces mouth ulcers, bleeding gums and excessive salivation.

Using the principle of *like cures like*, when we see a patient with sudden high fever, red flushed cheeks and dilated pupils we are led towards prescribing Belladonna, and when we see a patient with mouth ulcers, bleeding gums and excessive salivation, we look to Mercurius. The symptoms guide us to the remedy.

The remedies act by communicating with the body's own immune system, or vital life force. By producing these same symptoms, the remedy supports the organism's own chosen response to disease or disturbance. Sometimes the organism needs the additional stimulation produced by the most similar (similimum in Latin) remedy, to reset or support the immune response enabling it to complete its own action to combat the disturbance. The remedy supports and completes the action of the organism.

In his paper entitled, 'The Spin of Electrons and the Proof for the Action of Homeopathic Remedies',[6] Vithoulkas suggests this action may be the result of a change in the directional spin of the electron established during the process of succussion and potentiation of the remedy. You can read his published paper in the Journal of Medicine.

So, often when you take a remedy, you may experience an aggravation of symptoms. This is a sign that the remedy is correct because it further stimulates or resets the action of the organism. Ultimately the organism will do what it needs to do to survive, and the remedy supports that action.

Understanding the Aggravation

When a person ingests the raw plant Belladonna, the symptom produced as a reaction to the toxins in the plant are similar to those produced by a fast onset high fever, namely; dilated pupils, severe headache, delirium, convulsions, dry mouth, rash, fast heartbeat, flushed face, slurred speech, urine retention and hallucinations. So, when we give the diluted homeopathic remedy Belladonna to someone who has a fast onset high fever, the remedy helps by supporting the action of the organism to reach its goal; to quickly produce a high enough fever that will stimulate the immediate production of white blood cells to fight the infectious agent, to take the energy away from the peripheral towards the head.

The action of the organism is supported by the remedy, and if the organism is healthy enough, an amelioration of symptoms will naturally follow. This is why an aggravation is seen as a confirmation that the remedy is correct.

It is important to also understand that in vulnerable or elderly patients or those with complications or a weak disposition, we don't want that aggravation to be too intense. We also don't want to create a strong aggravation in certain conditions such as tuberculosis, eczema or asthma which would cause a lot of discomfort and put the organism at risk. So we

---

[6] The Spin of Electrons and the Proof for the Action of Homeopathic Remedies - Journal of Medicine and Life Vol. 13, Issue 3, July-September 2020, pp. 278–282

have to be careful not to give too high potencies, or to overstimulate by repeating the remedy too frequently.

Proving the Remedy

A sensitive and healthy volunteer may prove a remedy but so may a patient. When we give a close but not exact remedy the patient may express symptoms of the remedy which don't belong to the pathology of the disease. We don't need to worry too much about this because the symptoms will soon dissipate. They are expressions of the remedy and indicate a certain sensitivity of that organism to that particular remedy, which is why some will prove a remedy and others won't.

Also, when we give the correct remedy, we may see some symptoms of the remedy being expressed which were not there to begin with. For example, if you take the remedy Ipecacuanha for nausea during pregnancy, and then you get a strong pain between your shoulder blades which runs up into the back of your head, even though it wasn't there before, this is a side effect of the remedy and it will pass.

The Law of Cure

Herring's Law of Cure states that cure takes place in a certain order.
From above downwards, from within outwards, from the more important organs to the less important organs and in reverse order of their appearance.

From above downwards-

The general idea is that as the organism strengthens, it throws symptoms off towards the more superficial systems and layers of the body. So, we like to see the downward and outward movement of a disease in the form of a rash, hives, or a skin condition. Downwards meaning towards the extremities, the legs and then the feet, or hands.

From within, outwards-

An example of this may be a child who has an ongoing asthmatic cough, alleviated after the correct remedy. Then, a few months later the child develops a terrible runny nose attributed to seasonal allergies. For this again he is treated with the correct remedy. Finally, he gets a high fever followed by a rash. The disturbance started in the lungs, moved upwards and outwards into the nasal passages and finally out onto the skin in the form of a mild rash, with the help of a high fever.

From the more important organs to the less important organs-

On the physical level the most important organs, such as the brain and the heart, sit higher on the hierarchy of importance than the stomach or the skin.

Let's say we have a child who has a severe bronchial infection, with a very high fever. We understand that a very high and fast onset fever may cause convulsions which can be very dangerous. If we treat the child with the correct homeopathic remedy, the fever comes down. Now we are left with a child who has a thick mucus cough. After a few days we observe that the mucus has thickened and is drying up but now the child has diarrhea which lasts for a few days and then the child recovers fully. This is the correct direction of cure- from the most important organ-the brain, to a somewhat less important organ- the lungs, to a lesser important organ, the stomach and digestive tract.

This hierarchy applies equally to the emotional and mental cognitive bodies. On the emotional level a deep depression in which one is tempted to take one's life, is more critical than irritability. On the mental level, a complete breakdown of the mental faculties, where a patient may forget how to feed themselves, is more threatening than simple carelessness. Later we will see how illness expresses itself in all the bodies simultaneously and what that tells us about the movement towards healing. (See chapter 5- A deeper Understanding, Direction of Cure within a Complex Organism).

From the Mental to the Emotional to the Physical-

We like to see the movement from the mental to the emotional to the physical bodies as the mental faculty is higher in the order of importance. A child who is showing symptoms of ritualistic behaviors, might, after the correct remedy, stop lining up their toys and start expressing a deep sadness. After a period of emotional release, crying every day for a few weeks, the child might get a very sore throat with inflammation of the tonsils and a high fever. If the parents don't treat with antibiotics at this point, there is a good chance that the child will be quite well after he or she recovers from the physical discharge as the tonsils become puss-filled and suppurate, especially if in the past this was suppressed.

In reverse order of their appearance-

The mother may then remember that after the first course of antibiotics, the child started having tantrums, and then the ritualistic behavior started because often we see a reverse order of symptoms, especially if symptoms have been suppressed.

Another example may be when we treat inflamed tonsils we may find, and indeed we will be very happy to find that old ear infections return. As the organism gains strength, it is able to retrace its own line of defense before symptoms were suppressed. The old symptoms will usually be less severe and pass quicker than when they first appeared. It is here that the challenge lies for parents not to resort to suppressive medications or even acute homeopathic treatments which may also be suppressive.

CHAPTER 3

Treatments

The part can never be well, unless the whole is well.

Plato

Homeopathy looks to understand the physical, emotional and cognitive/mental health of the patient as well as their vitality.

Always remember that when we look for a remedy, we are focused on pathology and not on personality. Your highly spirited little one will probably always be somewhat demanding and your shy one will probably always be a little timid. Homeopathy will strengthen them both to be better adjusted in the world, but their personality is not what we aim to change.

When looking for a remedy match, we look for a remedy which covers the immediate, **acute, physical symptoms** such as- cough, as well as some **descriptive features** about the acute symptoms such as- dry, barking, hacking, and we look for **modalities**, meaning things that make the condition and the patient better or worse. For example, cough worse for lying down, or cough better with hot drinks.

Then we look for some **general physical symptoms** such as thirsty for small sips, chilly, some **emotional symptoms** such as desires company, aggravated while alone and some **mental symptoms** such as fastidious. This gives us a more well-rounded picture.

We look for a **totality of symptoms** by including all symptoms from all systems. You can run through a checklist from top to tail: head, eyes, ears, nose, throat, neck, shoulders, armpits, arms, upper chest, lungs etc. and see if there's anything you may have missed. Nothing should be excluded. So even if your child has this dry, barking cough and a concave chest since birth, even though it may seem unimportant, you will see when you check your symptoms against a remedy that this information may be a deciding factor in your remedy choice.

Sometimes we just have to settle for treating symptoms but sometimes we strike gold and are able to match more than just local symptoms and this is when deep changes take place. For example, if a child with a stomach bug is shivery, with burning pains, diarrhea and/or vomiting and is thirsty for small sips of water, you could give Arsenicum. But if that same child is also often anxious about his health, fastidious and critical about himself and others and likes the security of someone being around, you can be certain that Arsenicum will act, and it will act deeply. You would be treating the acute with a deep acting constitutional remedy because the child fits the remedy on all levels, physical, emotional and mental.

However, if you only have a few physical symptoms and not much else, which is often the case with little ones, you can still find a good remedy match by observing the symptoms well.

Constitutional Treatment

A constitutional treatment means the homeopath will take a full case history, including family history of disease, birth history, and disease history. We will look for a remedy which best matches the current symptoms, on all levels, and we will observe the temperament and nature of the patient. We also look for peculiarities of the case and causative factors. Constitutional remedies should not be given by parents, unless the remedy picture is very clear. A confused remedy picture can be difficult to sort through, even for the most experienced homeopath.

Constitutions change over time, the same way we do. It's rare to have one constitutional remedy your whole life, especially today. But in a healthy person, a constitutional remedy can often be used to ward off an acute if caught early enough. If you know your child's constitutional remedy, and they develop a sore throat, repeating a dose of their current constitutional remedy, (if the symptoms are included in the remedy description) may nip it in the bud. But please discuss with your homeopath first because an acute episode, following a constitutional treatment means something important.

Chronic Treatment

Chronic health issues should be treated by certified classical homeopaths. These might include: chronic lumbago (back ache), migraines, digestive problems, seasonal and/or chronic allergies, hay-fever, asthma, eczema, ulcers, warts, skin conditions, colitis, gastritis, sinusitis, rhinitis, cystitis, bronchitis, idiopathic hypertension, hormonal imbalances, chronic fatigue, hyperactivity, AD/HD, collagen diseases, arthritis, neuromuscular diseases, degenerative diseases and heart, kidney or liver diseases.

Acute Treatments

PHYSICAL

Mostly, you will be treating your family at home for acute physical symptoms. These may include; teething pain, coughs, colds, viruses, inflammation of the mucous membranes- runny or blocked nose, sore throats, inflamed tonsils, ear infections, upper respiratory infections, minor burns, cuts, blunt instrument wounds- bumps and bruises, fevers, stomach bugs, sore muscles, growing pains, muscle cramps, menstrual cramps, eye infections, bites and stings, cuts, wounds, headaches, toothache, diarrhea, constipation, vomiting, worms, stomach bugs and the symptoms associated with common childhood diseases- chicken pox, measles, whooping cough, etc.

Teething babies can be hard to deal with, especially if they keep you and themselves up all night. If they are in a great deal of pain, cranky, throwing down the toy they just demanded and generally miserable, look at **Chamomilla.** Chamomilla babies are very sensitive to pain and just want to be carried. They will scream blue murder if you try put them down and they cannot be soothed. Often one cheek or one ear will be red, which may also indicate otitis (ear infections, which Chamomilla can treat well). **Pulsatilla** babies will present with yellow or green mucous and will be very clingy too, but they are generally milder in nature that Chamomilla babes.

Fevers are a natural and important part of healthy immune expression and should not be suppressed with medication. If your child is very uncomfortable and the fever seems to be taking its toll or climbing rapidly, there are some natural measures you can take to bring it down. Soak a cloth in a vinegar to water dilution 1:6, squeeze out the liquid and place the cloth on the back of the neck, forehead or soles of the feet drawing the fever down and out. You can also use cabbage leaves on the feet to do the same. Cold cabbage leaves will also help cool down engorged breasts. Replace them when they get limp and warm- the leaves, not the breasts ;)

You can also bathe the child in a tepid to warm bath to cool them down. Make sure the water is not too cold and as soon as they start to cool down take them out, dry them well and dress in cotton or natural fiber clothes. Of course, do this in a temperature-controlled environment. **Belladonna** is one of the first but certainly not the only fever remedy. The Belladonna fever comes up fast, the picture is hot, red, dry and throbbing. The **Ferrum-phos** fever is slower to come on and has the associated upper respiratory inflammation of common colds and flues.

Acute **Stomach bugs** should last no more than 24-48 hours and usually respond well to homeopathy. **Arsenicum, Nux-vomica** and **Lycopodium** are the first remedies to look at if symptoms match. Arsenicum is chilly, restless and feel like they have been poisoned. Nux-Vomica is better suited for overindulgence or eating too much of the wrong foods. The **BRAT** diet (Banana, Rice, Apple and Toast) can be followed during bouts of diarrhea and/or vomiting. Often fevers accompany vomiting but if your child is well hydrated, responsive and passing a normal amount of urine, you can treat stomach bugs at home. If your child refuses to drink, be creative- a sick child may agree to an iced fruit popsicle, to suck on ice-cubes or to drink juice through a fancy straw. Herb teas may be tolerated and diluted apple juice 1:7 is easy on the stomach. Watch out for signs of dehydration as children dehydrate very fast.

Ears can be kept wax free with ear-candles which create a gentle vacuum sucking out build-up of wax. Make a calm space and lie your child flat on their side in a quiet room. You may prop a flat pillow under their head. Place the candle in their ear holding it gently till it burns down to the marked safety line. Children love to hear the crackling of the wax and having some special time and attention. They also love to see what comes out at the end. You can cut the solid plastic end tube open to see, you will be pleasantly surprised at your child's waxy deposits.

If your little one suffers from ear infections, there are many remedies you can look at but if it is chronic, it's best to consult with a practitioner. Pain in the ears which comes on suddenly after exposure to cold winds can sometimes be nipped in the bud with a dose of **Aconite** if caught early. The ear may be hot and red, with throbbing, cutting pain. **Calc-carb** can also present throbbing pain with swollen glands and pain on blowing the nose. Calc-carb children love sweet milky foods, eggs and usually sweat behind their neck during sleep. **Pulsatilla** earaches have throbbing, stitching pains, are worse at night, with thick yellow-green discharge. The outer ear can be red and often one cheek is red too.

Minor burns can be immediately placed in cold salted water and treated with **Cantharis** or **Causticum** when symptoms match. **Growing Pains** and **tics** can be treated with magnesium supplements, which also helps relieve muscle pains. Growing pains may also be an indication for homeopathic **Phosphorous** in children who grow too quickly.

Years ago, when my children were very young, we lived in a rainforest in Australia. I remember the long drive into town, through winding dirt roads and creek crossings finally arriving at the clearing which lead us into Australia's largest small town, Mullumbimby. The health food co-op was full of colorful characters many of whom lived up in the forest. Next to the health food store was a sweet little herbalist who made up tinctures and potions. For years, every time we came to visit that old hippy town, I would stock up on a bottle of **Ledum tincture**. Nothing treated the itch of a nasty bite as effectively as a few drops of Ledum. To this day my adult children still ask for it when they itch.

Ledum and **Apis** are the go-to remedies for **insect bites and stings**. Apis is made from bee venom, and will bring down hot, red inflamed swellings, where the Ledum wound is cold. Ledum is also used for puncture wounds.

EMOTIONAL

As parents, you will also be called on to deal with acute emotional symptoms such as: temper tantrums, night terrors, pre-menstrual moodiness, sadness and grief, all kinds of fears; of the known, of the unknown and of the imagined- storms, lightening, thunder, nightmares, dogs, cats, dark, insects, stings, heights, closed spaces, crowds, open spaces, performance anxiety, and general anxiety in young children and teens. Please note that if your child has been damaged by vaccinations, they should be treated by a professional homeopath and I recommend a functional doctor who can order the correct tests and look for specific deficiencies. Ultimately, I believe vaccine damaged children will have to undergo some form of chelation if metals are the culprit.

The Great Catastrophe Scale

The human brain doesn't stop developing until we are well into young adult life, and since we ourselves are such reactive and emotional beings, managing our children's emotional outbursts can be extremely challenging. Here's a little trick esteemed Sydney psychologist Renee Mill taught me when my children were young.

Draw the numbers from 1 to 10 on a piece of colored paper and stick it on the fridge. This is a Catastrophe Scale. When your child experiences a seeming catastrophe, ask them to place the event on the scale.

You can help with some example. Losing your favorite hair clip or not getting ice-cream might be a one or a two. Crashing your bike and scraping your knee might be a five, breaking a limb might be a seven, and maybe something really terrible like losing a beloved grandparent might be a nine, whereas being displaced by war or famine, would be a ten. You can discuss different examples with them as they arise, asking your child where they might place the event on the scale.

In times of crisis (or perceived crisis) or during meltdowns, you can ask your child, what number is this on the catastrophe scale? This will help them rate their emotional losses and disappointments more realistically giving them perspective and emotional control over their own response to 'disaster'.

Fright and Grief

When parents ask for a remedy for a child who has had a minor fright or one going through the natural grieving process after the loss of a loved one or animal, or the severing of a friendship, I usually advise them to use Bach Flower remedies. I find Rescue remedy to be very useful when the grief is natural, and the response is healthy, albeit upsetting. Grief is a natural and healthy response to loss and should not be interfered with if it is not pathological.

Rituals are a good way for children to manage grief. They can write a letter, keep a journal, send a blessing to the deceased in a sky lantern, light a candle, engrave the name of the lost person or animal on a bracelet or pendant, burry an associated article, paint or draw an image and hang it in their room, or frame a special photograph. Remembering our ancestors is important for family constellation health and parents need to be able to hold children in their grief without freaking out themselves. If their grief triggers your own, seek homeopathic support or grief counselling.

Some children are very sensitive to hearing bad news or frightening or violent stories. Share this information with your homeopath as it is important. You can protect these children to a certain extent, but at some point, they will probably hear about something they find too much for their little psyche to manage and they may start playing out or sobbing, wetting the bed at night, regressing, waking from nightmares, or they may withdraw. It's important that they have a safe place to speak about whatever they have heard or experienced. Enquire gently using reflective listening skills. *How to Talk So Kids Will Listen and Listen So Kids Will Talk*,[7] is an excellent book on effective communication and reflective listening skills.

When is grief considered pathology? Grief is pathological when despair sets in and interferes with the normal day-to- day running of our lives. In the Jewish tradition, following the death of an immediate family member, seven days of mourning are set aside, where the immediate family remain in the family home, and visitors come to pay their respects and comfort the mourners. This is followed by a thirty-day mark, then a one-year mark and then an annual memorial ritual, either visiting the grave, lighting a long burning candle, or sharing a family meal. This marking of a defined time allows for the healthy integration of the mourner, back into daily life. When a child loses a beloved grandparent, a best friend, a pet, a home, or a parent through divorce or separation, you can help them navigate the loss through a ritual marking of the loss.

---

[7] Adele Faber, Elaine Mazlish - 'How to talk so Kids will Listen and Listen so Kids will Talk'

If they lose their appetite, shut themselves in their room, don't cry or express any emotions, shut down, cry continuously, can't sleep because of intrusive thoughts, have repetitive thoughts, repeated bad dreams or nightmares and of course any ideas of self-harm or running away, a professional homeopath or therapist should be consulted.

There are specific **remedies for fright,** such as **Stramonium** for night terrors. Often a child will only need one dose of Stramonium once and the night terrors will become a thing of the past. It is really miraculous and quite unbelievable to watch. Stramonium has won over many a doubtful partner to Homeopathy.

Aconite is a good remedy for panic attacks. When the person is overcome with a real sense of panic with all the accompanying physiological symptoms- increased pulse, cold sweat, shortness of breath and a sense that they are in real danger, even if they know they are not. This may happen during a flight or in a claustrophobic environment, in a crowd or a narrow space. If a patient has post-traumatic stress disorder (PTSD), Aconite can help settle the panic attack in the moment, but a classical homeopath should be consulted for long term care. Panic attacks can happen after an emotional shock or realization. And of course, one of the keynotes, is sudden onset. So, if a child suddenly comes down with a high fever, or sore throat, especially after exposure to cold/winds, often you can nip it in the bud with a dose of Aconite.

Grief remedies tend to be for the emotionally sensitive types. **Ignatia** suffers terribly from lost love, whether it be a partner, a lover, a best friend, a crush, or the parent of the opposite sex. There is a romantic nature to the patient and/or the relationship. Grown women who lose their beloved fathers often need Ignatia as much as their teenage daughters who weep silently in their rooms because their crush is ghosting them on social media. Ignatia is delicate, sensitive, creative, artistic. They take everything to heart, and do not do well with romantic disappointments. You will hear long sighs and observe some difficulty catching a full breath. They will join the family for dinner, but their grief will show through and even though they are devastated, they will usually cry alone. A dose of Ignatia will change their entire countenance in a few days.

Nat-mur is a more serious and deep acting grief remedy. They are more closed, private, and will only break down under extreme circumstances or with one or two people. But the grief runs deep. Perhaps there was emotional trauma during childbirth or even during the pregnancy. Perhaps there was a deep loss, or the child was separated from his mother and denied immediate contact with her for whatever reason. Or perhaps there was a series of losses and griefs which settled deep in the organism. Nat-mur salt their food well (the expression 'salting an open wound' comes to mind), and they suffer in the heat from headaches. It's also a good remedy for violent nasal symptoms- a running nose with sneezing which accompanies a head cold and is followed by thick mucus which sets in obstructing breathing.

MENTAL & COGNITIVE

There will also be some acute mental symptoms which will be equally as challenging. These include apathy, absent mindedness, forgetfulness, lack of focus and concentration, forgetting words, incorrect writing, stammering, confusion. Many mental health or learning disabilities can be corrected if caught early enough. Mental issues must be treated by a qualified homeopath as they are the deepest level of disturbance.

Nutritional deficiencies are often the cause of learning and cognitive issues. Few of us have enough zinc in our diets because the earth is so depleted of nutrients and zinc is essential for healthy brain function. Many of us are also depleted of the B vitamins, and now with the fear of sunshine which has slowly been indoctrinated into, many are depleted of vitamin D.

A thorough blood test and hair analysis will show deficiencies in vitamins and minerals. You can work with an integrative doctor or naturopath to bring these back into balance. You will see your child's mental and cognitive functions improve as well as their ability to handle stress if their nutritional needs are taken care of. Long gone are the days when your doctor's advice to follow 'a balanced diet', was enough for our children's dietary needs. Today, we need to be extra vigilant and follow a vitamin-nutrient rich and probiotic-high diet.

Preventative Treatment

Some Homeopaths treat using homeo-prophylaxis (HP)- a system of administering homeopathic doses of a nosode (a homoeopathically diluted infectious pathogen), such as Pertussis for Whooping Cough. Dr Isaac Golden published a Fifteen-year Study, which showed a 90% effectiveness rate for preventing pertussis amongst the children in his study and showed good long term health outcomes.

During pandemics, a general widely distributed 'genus epidemicus' may be effective in protecting large portions of the population. For example, in 2007, during an outbreak of leptospirosis in Cuba, a homeopathic remedy mix was distributed to two and a half million people. "Cases of leptospirosis increased by 27% on the island, apart from in the 3 intervened provinces, where rates of infection reduced by 84% The epidemic was halted within two weeks and the levels of this disease dropped far below the historical averages for years afterwards. The report concluded: The homeo-prophylactic approach was associated with a large reduction of disease incidence and control of the epidemic."[8]

Generally speaking, homeo-prophylaxis is not used by classical homeopaths who rely on presenting symptoms.

---

[8] https://magicpillsmovie.com/cuba-the-country-that-dares-to-be-wise/?fbclid=IwAR3yke0Ixq48QVzhwnGXwG6_N-6bGMwv6oX6WjsbW03b32fwx_UTwt_-hHA

CHAPTER 4

Finding the remedy

A women's psychic tasks are these: learning fine discrimination, separating one thing from the other with finest discernment, learning to make fine distinctions in judgement.

Clasrissa Pinkola Estes

How do we match the remedy when there are so many to choose from and so many symptoms in each remedy description? It can be overwhelming. The first thing to remember is that you don't have to match all the symptoms listed under each remedy, you only have to match the ones relevant to your patient.

Each remedy has an essential nature, an individual energetic imprint, a frequency. As you come to familiarize yourself with the homeopathic literature, it will become clearer and easier to identify the essence of a remedy and match it to the essential expression of the disease, and then with time and practice, you will be able to match it to the essential expression of your child during different periods of their life.

Rudolf Steiner, creator of the anthroposophical philosophies which include the Waldorf education system, divided children's developmental progress into three main periods and ages. The general movement being from limitation (birth to seven) through imagination (seven to fourteen) and on towards authority (fourteen to twenty-one); from the development of the will to the feeling state to the development of abstract thought. At each transition we observe a kind of shedding of the old self, as the child steps into the challenges of the new, and we see this similar process in homeopathy, where a constitution sheds to reveal a new layer.

It may be physical as they grow adult teeth or recover from a childhood disease. It may be emotional as they process complex feelings and mature with a deeper understanding of themselves and their relationships, or it may be in the mental realm as they push themselves to meet a learning challenge building and strengthening the powers of the mind. As one layer falls away a new one emerges with its own complexities and process.

Putting the Pieces Together

Here is an acronym you can use to remember what to look for, to more easily identify symptoms and help guide you towards finding the correct remedy.

Sensation, Influence, Cause and Keynote, or SICK.

Sensation in this context is not a reference to The Sensation Method taught by Sankaran.

Sensation.

Many physical symptoms are described by patients using the word "pain". Pain is a general term used to describe many forms of discomfort. But if you really tune in to the affected area you will begin to notice that there are many different sensations. A scraped knee has a particular sting to it, a urinary tract infection burns, a strained muscle aches, a headache pounds or pulsates, a sinus infection creates pressure, a gallstone radiates. I encourage you to refine your search terms.

Sensation Meditation

The cure for the pain is in the pain - Rumi

I like to introduce children (and parents) to this sensation meditation, which will serve as an invaluable tool throughout their lives. First, replace the word 'pain' with the words 'sensations' or 'feelings. Ask your loved one to close their eyes and focus their attention on the area of concern. Then ask them to describe the sensation they feel without using the words 'pain', 'painful' or 'sore'. Ask them, is the area warm or cool? Is the sensation sharp, stabbing, dull or throbbing? Does it stay in one place or does it move? Does it have a shape? Does it have edges? Does it have a color? Is it tight like a band, or does it flow? Is it crushing, or smarting? Is it tingling or numb? Does it pulsate or is it pounding, like little hammers? Does it have a sound? Does it feel swollen? Is it itchy? Is it dry?

By focusing in this way, instead of resisting the pain, and creating tension around it, we enter into it and really feel it, almost like a meditation. This allows us to better manage pain during acute and chronic events. It can also be used as a powerful tool during labor.

Influence

What influences the condition (or the patient), making the sensation (or the patient) better or worse? What are the modalities? Does your little one want to be wrapped up warm and snuggly, resting quietly close to you, or are they better with the window flung wide open, in their underwear lying under a fan? Do they want to drink warm tea or suck on cubes of ice? Do they want the shutters closed and the room quiet? Do they want to be alone and not move much or are they restless, going from the sofa to the bed? Are they thirsty, if so for small sips or big gulps? For warm drinks or for iced ones? Do they want attention, affection, reassurance, or are they best left alone?

In the list of remedies (in the Repertory), under modalities for each remedy, you will see the description of symptoms as worse and/or better. They are often indicated with these signs: < meaning worse from   > meaning better from.

For example: **Hepar-sulph**, which may be used to treat infected tonsils which feel like splinters in the throat, is **better from >** warmth, >a warm room, >wet weather and >after a meal. They are **worse from <** cool air, <the cold, <winter, <cold dry winds, <a draught, <cold foods or drinks, <any kind of touch, <mornings and evenings. These modalities help us differentiate one remedy from another.

Cause

The 'exciting' cause helps us to prescribe because it points to a vulnerability in the organism, or a point during which the organism was set off course (stressed), and this can help lead us in a remedy choice. An obvious example may be a sting from an insect, which will lead us to a select from a few remedies such as Apis, Ledum, Urtica Urens. The exciting cause may be from an emotional upset, which will guide us towards a different set of remedies, the grief remedies like Ignatia, Nat.Mur or Aurum. Or the exciting cause could be something like 'never well since': vaccination, or the Chicken Pox, or since falling off a skate-board, and again we are directed towards a specific group of remedies, perhaps Arnica, Gelsemium or Nat-Sulph.

Start to become aware of the exciting cause of your own ailments. If you have severe menstrual cramps, perhaps they started after the birth of a child. If your partner has bursitis, perhaps it started after he began taking medication for a different problem. If your little one is suddenly anxious and wetting himself at night after being dry for a year, explore what was happening at the time in the family, in his social environment, at school etc. How did it begin? Did the cough start after a late afternoon baseball game when the autumn winds picked up unexpectedly? Or after a long day in the hot summer sun? Was there an emotional upset? A rejection by a friend or group of friends, or a nasty remark made by someone considered important? Ask your child too. Sometimes they remember things we know nothing about. "Yes, I started to get stomach cramps after dad took me for a burger to cheer me up after practice, because I didn't make the team," they may say, or, "I remember feeling better before went on our camping trip".

Keynotes

Keynotes are modalities which are specific to remedies and are also peculiar. **Nat-Mur** will take a potato wedge and dip it right into the salt bowl. **Medorrhinum** can't walk on a pebbled beach, the soles of the feet are so very sensitive. The feet of **Sulphur** get so hot at night that they are found sticking out the covers, and **Calc-carb** sweats so much at the back of their head that the pillow is damp in the morning.

Peculiarities alert us to something unusual about the case. They help us confirm remedy choices. For example, **Sulphur** gets ravenously hungry mid-morning. Remember the Hobbits mid-morning meal, this is a typical Sulphur peculiarity. They also find it difficult to stand for any length of time. They will be the first to lie down on a comfortable couch or fling themselves over an armchair regardless of their social surroundings. As a young teen, my Sulphur boyfriend would come over and lay himself comfortably across the sofa and when my parents came home, he would not get up or even sit up to say hello. Another peculiarity may be a teenage boy who feels compelled to stick his knife into the toaster even though he knows it's dangerous. This is peculiar, and it points to a keynote of **Argentum-nitricum** who are highly impulsive, sometimes stupidly so.

Now that you have something of a picture, think about the child, and collect some general symptoms. In what position do they sleep? Do they run hot or cold? What are their favorite types of foods? Are they extroverted or introverted, inquisitive wanting to know how things work or more social? Are they selfish and critical or sympathetic and caring? What is their nature? Though we never treat personality, temperament can help direct us.

Differentiating

Sometimes it's hard to differentiate between remedies because many of the bigger remedies cover so many different physical pathologies. Sulphur, Phosphorous, Lycopodium, Cal Carb all have long lists of symptoms and many cover the same symptoms, so you have to learn to discern between some of the subtle points. There is some detective work involved. You have to investigate well and learn to differentiate. For example:

Nux-vomica and **Arsenicum** both have diarrhea from the slightest indiscretion in eating, digestive complaints and ulcers. They are both aggravated by the cold and cold foods and they are both anxious remedies, but their personalities are quite different. **Arsenicum** is really anxious about his health, he worries a lot. He is a hypochondriacal and every small health concern is exaggerated in his mind. He has an aversion to foods, especially greasy foods. But he is milder than Nux-vom. **Nux-vomica** is a domineering type, argumentative, controlling, easily angered and easily irritated. Nux-vomica loves to indulge in tasty, spices, highly seasoned foods and he loves stimulants, but he suffers from them.

We see here two remedies with very similar pathology details, but quite different pictures. Both suffer from digestive complaints and from the cold, both are anxious and fastidious, both prefer hot drinks and warm food but Arsenicum creates order (because the chaos of the unknown unnerves him) and makes attachments to feel secure (because he is sure he is going to die and needs someone to be with him in case anything happens), where Nux-vomica demands order, the way he wants it, and he likes to be in control. He is more domineering, stronger, has more authority. These differences help us to choose one remedy over another.

With babies and infants, differentiating is harder, so in acute situations, I advise parents to try a remedy they believe matches well in a low potency. If, after an hour or two you don't observe any change, move on to the other remedy. It's best not to do this too often or to treat with too many remedies. The general rule in homeopathy is to wait and give the organism time to adjust. You will have to use your own sense of intuition coupled with common sense or find a homeopath with whom you can communicate easily and ask for direction. Eventually you will get the hang of it.

For the Womenfolk

Intuition is not something we rely on in homeopathy, but it is definitely a muscle we should exercise as mothers. You can practice exercising it by listening to your inner voice. You know, the one that tells you to buy the pasta in the supermarket, or wait for the parking spot, or check your bank account, or call your sister. The more we listen to that voice, the clearer she will become. Nobody knows your child as well as you. The stronger your intuitive muscle becomes, the more you will be able to voice your deepest knowing about what is best for your child at any given moment. It is usually fear that allows us to give in to the voice of an authority we neither know nor completely trust and we are the ones that end up paying. The psychology behind sales and marketing is built on undermining your intuition as a mother and a woman and influencing you not to trust yourself and therefore depend on the 'safety', 'security' and 'fantasy' of whatever is being sold. It is a trick, don't fall for it. You are smarter than that.

For young mothers looking to understand the traps and pitfalls and to strengthen yourself psychically and emotionally I recommend you read *Women Who Run with the Wolves,* by Clarissa Pinkola Estes. It is a brilliant book, and I cannot recommend it highly enough. We have lost touch with our grounded, earth connected power as women, and we are now going into the fourth and fifth generations of disempowered women which is a deep tragedy for motherhood and for womanhood. Some of us still have a grandmother dancing around the fire, but I imagine that is rare. For the most part you will find her trusting the pamphlet because it's so slick and printed on such expensive paper. If that's the case, it's time to reclaim your wild woman. The sooner you do it the better, your daughters will thank you, and your sons will be attracted to wild protective and intuitive women who will not be afraid to stand their ground and protect your grand babies.

Do not be put off by the word 'wild'. Wild does not mean without religion, without sacred connection to God or morality. In fact, it means quite the opposite. It means wild enough to say NO, at the right time and to the right things, and wild enough to say YES at the right time and to the right things, and intuitive enough to know the difference, regardless of social pressure and expectations.

CHAPTER 5

A Deeper Understanding

The long-term benefits of Homeopathy to the patient is that it not only alleviates the presenting symptoms but it reestablishes internal order at the deepest levels and thereby provides a lasting cure.

George Vithoulkas

When you first come across homeopathy, it seems so simple and very exciting, but it is also very complicated and easy to get tangled up in if you don't understand what master Homeopath, George Vithoulkas refers to as, *correct homeopathic prescribing*. This chapter is to introduce parents to some of the more complex theories of homeopathy (and specifically to the teachings of George Vithoulkas), so they will be better equipped to treat their own families well.

Homeopathy is not just about matching symptoms to remedies and giving your children Arnica every-time they bump their heads; it is much more complicated than that- we are much more complicated than that.

Building on the principles of the masters, Hahnemann, Boericke, Herring and Kent, George Vithoulkas introduced and established some groundbreaking ideas, not just to homeopathy but to medicine as well. His theories on Levels of Health and the Continuum of Disease, are studied in depth by doctors who come from across the globe to learn from the master at his Academy of Classical Homeopathy, in Alonnisos, Greece. They have won him international acclaim and honorary titles from numerous Medical institutions the world over. His theories are well beyond the scope of this book, but I will introduce some of the ideas which I hope will help parents better understand treatment protocols.

Layers

We already understand that the patient throws out symptoms and the symptoms guide us towards the correct remedy. But what if our little patient has some matching symptoms but not all, or when specific symptoms don't match the remedy? Or when the emotional and mental symptoms match but there are no physical symptoms or visa-versa.

A child may be typically **Sulphur**. They may be hot and grubby, fiercely independent and full of fascinating conversation and theories, they may put the shoes on the wrong feet and their dress on backwards and wipe their grubby hands all over their clothes and pull things apart just to see how they work, oblivious to the chaos they leave behind them. They may be thirsty, curious and very bright. They may love sweets and also love soft boiled eggs. But typically, Sulphur has an aversion to eggs. Would we still give this child Sulphur even with this keynote, **aversion to eggs?** It's confusing.

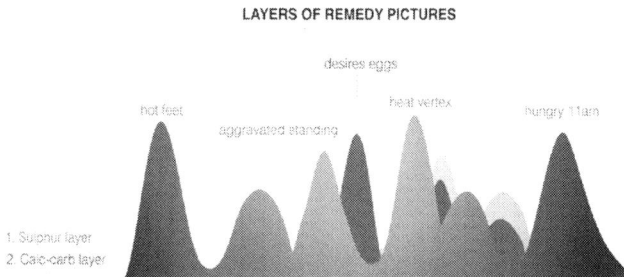

LAYERS OF REMEDY PICTURES

If the symptoms match, and the essence of the child fits the essence of the remedy, we can still give the remedy even if one or two keynotes do not belong. The keynote which doesn't fit the remedy may indicate a strong feature of an underlying remedy layer. So, if your little Sulphur child has red swollen tonsils, you can treat them with a single dose of Sulphur, even if they like eggs. What you will probably find, after some time, is that the Sulphur layer will clear and the picture of the next layer, probably Calc-carb, who do love eggs, will develop.

Now after some time, you may find your previously hot Sulphur child has quite a few fears and cold feet, a love of rich creamy deserts, and the pillow on which she sleeps is damp from sweating behind the head during sleep.

Symptoms

The defense mechanism generates a specific set of symptoms as a response to specific stress and stimuli. Vithoulkas.

The defense mechanism knows what it needs to do to save the organism. In the case of an infection, the brain may signal the thermostat to raise a temperature to increases the production of white fighter blood cells (T-cells- leukocytes). Inflammation, increased production of mucous and increased circulation are other ways an organism may respond to a specific stress stimulus in an attempt to save itself.

Crying or talking incessantly, may be ways an organism responds 'emotionally' to a specific stress stimulus. Whatever the response, it must be observed and respected. We must ask, how is the organism trying to heal itself? What is it trying to do? And then we follow its lead.

In homeopathy, we respect the symptoms of the patient and we work to support those symptoms, trusting the innate wisdom of a healthy defense mechanism. We should never underestimate the importance of an immune response which can still raise a fever and we should not suppress the fever unless it is life threatening or harmful. For the most part, the danger of a high fever has more to do with the speed of onset which can cause cerebral inflammation. But generally, a fever is a VERY IMPORTANT indication of a healthy and strong immune system and should be left to run its course wherever possible. Today, with the widespread use of vaccinations and chemical drugs used across multiple generations, we have interfered too much with nature's immune system. There is much work to be done to restore good health

Progress of Disease

The symptoms show the path that the defense mechanism choses to counteract the disease. Vithoulkas

In Homeopathy, we understand that there is a specific series of responses, a path or the organism takes to manage disorder. Usually, the organism creates an acute inflammation as its first response to invasion. When the chosen path is repeatedly suppressed, (even across generations), the organism has no choice but to change tactics in dealing with the disturbance, eventually pushing it deeper into the system until it becomes chronic.

For example, if your child was repeatedly prescribed antibiotics for recurrent ear infections during the first year of her life, and then later developed chronic anxiety, we see these two symptoms as being connected. So during the treatment for the anxiety, if the old symptoms of the previously suppressed ear infections return, parents should understand that this is part of the restorative process and not rush to suppress the acute expression.

Chronic cases are complicated and should only be treated by a qualified practitioner who will be able to manage the often-precarious balance, as they step their patients back towards better health. In some cases, interfering with homeopathy can exacerbate an already too-fragile balance.

Direction of Cure within a Complex Organism

We already understand that with the correct treatment and according to Herring's Law of Cure, a healthy organism will move the disturbance from the most important to the least important organs and systems. But this movement can also flow between levels and systems, because we are holistic creatures. So, we may find that as the bronchial infection clears, the anxiety increases. Then we treat the anxiety and the sleeplessness increases, we treat the insomnia and old eczema returns.

Sometimes the emotional situation will improve but the physical symptoms will get worse. Then the physical symptoms will improve, and the emotional symptoms will get worse. As long as they are getting worse on a lower level on the hierarchy, we are managing the case well. As you can see it is quite complicated to gauge the progress of a case. So often, especially in chronic or constitutional care, it can be confusing, and progress looks elusive. With time (often years) and the correct sequence of remedies, the organism can return to an optimum state of health.

Levels of Health

Each of us is born with a potential longevity which correlates with our potential level of health. If we encounter high stress, if we make bad dietary and lifestyle choices, if we learn and model poor relationship patterns, if we pollute ourselves with chemicals and pharmaceutical drugs and vaccines, or if we are simply unlucky and encounter shock, accidents or trauma, we risk dropping our level of health and shortening our potential longevity.

A very healthy person will present a clear remedy picture, and will respond to the correct remedy quickly, often without an aggravation. As we go down in levels of health, we see more confused remedy pictures. We also see patients who are no longer able to amount a healthy immune response to disease. (This is why your homeopath will ask when you or your child last had a high fever.) In the lowest levels, homeopathy will only provide amelioration and assist in easy transitions.

The idea of levels of health is an important tool to understand the response of the organism to a remedy. And the response of the organism also tells us much about the level of health of the patient. Parents shouldn't get too caught up in trying to work out their child's level of health, but it gives us an insight into the complications practitioners face when making remedy and potency choices and it explains why some cases are so simple to treat while others present ongoing challenges.

Suppression of Symptoms

Give me a fever and I can cure the child.

Hippocrates

When we suppress the body's response to disease, we negatively affect our level of health. For example, one of a child's first lines of defense against invading pathogens, is her tonsils-those two gates at the back of the throat which swell up every time she gets sick. She suffers miserably, crying out during the night and finally her parents take her to the doctor who prescribes antibiotics. After two weeks she recovers, but two months later, again, she presents with the same symptoms, for which antibiotics are prescribed.

By the time the child is three she may have taken enough antibiotics to deplete her digestive tract of healthy gut bacteria, leaving her general overall immune system in quite bad shape. By now, the glands which line the digestive tract, are hard at work to constantly fight bacteria and the whole glandular system (including the tonsils) is too weak to put up a good fight. The infection now slips straight past the tonsils and heads down the bronchial tubes where the bacteria take up residence causing a persistent cough.

Consistent suppression of symptoms forces the organism to take the disturbance deeper. The job of the homeopath is to track and support the reversal of this process, respecting each step in the journey, until finally the child gets sick with swollen glands, inflamed tonsils and a high fever. If the parents are brave enough to nurse their child through, with natural treatments which support the body, on recovery, they will find an overall improvement in their child's vital health.

The correct remedy or sequence of remedies can help the organism retrace the steps it wanted to take in the first place to manage the disturbance in the best way it knew how, before it was suppressed. I am always excited when my patients tell me they or their children have a high fever, especially if they have not had one for a few years.

Hereditary (miasmic) Predispositions

As parents we do our best for our children's health, taking care of everything we consume throughout our pregnancy and nursing years. Most of us continue to make wholesome lifestyle choices to ensure the wellbeing and good health of our families. Yet sometimes, unfortunately, our kids are still sick and often, through no fault of our own. Years before scientists knew anything about genetics, homeopaths understood that hereditary predispositions influence individual health. We call this a miasm or a miasmatic influence.

We may find a grandfather who suffered terrible allergic rhinitis. His daughter may have suffered from chronic eczema. It would come as no surprise to a homeopath to see her child suffer from bronchial weakness or asthma. This is why a good homeopath will always ask about the family health and hereditary predispositions.

It has well been well documented that we inherit more than the physical genetic coding for certain traits and diseases. Trauma is engraved into our genetic imprint as well.[9] A descendent of a holocaust survivor or the grandchild of a slave or war veteran can pass on trauma and grief, and the child of a parent with mental health issues may carry the genetic predisposition for a mental breakdown.

Part of homeopathic theory is the idea that during the course of the history of disease of mankind, there have been three significant periods during which disease imprints have established themselves and settled amongst masses of populations. But in the last hundred years, the miasms for disease has grown exponentially, leaving us with miasms for almost all the chronic diseases we encounter today.

The four founding miasms we come across in classical Homeopathy are the psoric, sycotic, syphilitic and tubercular miasms.

The **Psoric** predisposition leads to deficiency or inactivity. Hypofunctions, scant secretions, low immunity, itching eruptions and inflammation.

The **Sycotic** predisposition (from fig warts, not the psychological condition psychosis) leads to excess and hyperactivity. Overproduction, stones, warts, scar tissue, restlessness.

The **Syphilitic** predisposition leads to destructive and degenerative conditions- ulcers, acidic discharges, perversions, depressed and suicidal tendencies.

The **Tubercular** predisposition leads to a mix of (and changeability between) the deficiency of psora and the destructive element of syphilinum and a general break down of the organism. Allergies, lymphatic and glandular swellings and a tendency to excessive bleeding are Tubercular.

---

[9] https://www.sciencedaily.com/releases/2014/04/140413135953.htm - Hereditary trauma: Inheritance of traumas and how they may be mediated.

Sometimes, a homeopath will look for a miasm which may seem to be getting in the way of the organism responding to a remedy. For example, a child who suffers from a seasonal croupy cough, may need a Tubercular remedy. The father may have suffered terribly from asthma as a child and then we find the grandfather passed away from lung disease. The correct Tubercular remedy will clear this predisposition from the genetic line and we will find that the child will then respond well to the indicated remedy.

This whole process can take months because we have to first treat the miasm and then wait for a clear picture of the original remedy to return, if it returns at all. The Tubercular remedy may clear it completely. It's important for parents to understand this because it can be frustrating that your homeopath is treating your child for a disease he doesn't seem to have. However, if you examine the remedy well, you will find some keynotes and symptoms which have been detected and which indicate the miasmic remedy. Be patient.

Response to the Remedy

We usually start with low potencies and wait to assess the effect of the remedy. This gives us somewhere to go when the action of the remedy stops being effective. But we also don't want to create a strong aggravation in a weak organism. And there's also an idea that some organisms simply resonate better with certain potencies. Some of it is trial and error.

There is a comprehensive methodology for assessing the response to the remedy, which is beyond the scope of this book. An acute reaction any time from a few days to a week or even months after a remedy must be reported back to your homeopath so she may include this important event in her case notes and in the understanding of the case. It is an important indicator of the level of health of the patient

The Follow-up

While your homeopath may ask you to check in a few days or a week after an acute, a follow-up generally takes place about 1 month after a constitutional treatment and then monthly after that, depending on the case.

Your follow-up assessment is as important as your initial consultations. It is here that ALL the work of assessing the action of the remedy is done. Your response to the remedy gives your homeopath clues about your level of health and it is here that the next prescription or no prescription is made. More often than not, if the remedy is correct and your homeopath can see even the slightest movement in the right direction, you will be asked to wait and return in another month.

You may feel disappointed that you have not been given a remedy to take when you still have so many complaints. This is a western medicine perspective- the belief that we need to take a pill for each ailment, but it has little to do with the overall strengthening of the organism and the movement towards health. In fact, quite the opposite. The fact that you are asked to wait means the stimulation initiated by the remedy is still active. Please do not underestimate the work your homeopath is doing during this follow up assessment which is a crucial part of your treatment.

CHAPTER 6

Healing Takes Time

Do you have the patience to wait till your mud settles and the water is clear?

Tao Te Ching

We are organic creatures living in a complex biological environment. When we suffer a disturbance on any level, whether it be a paper cut or heartbreak, our chemistry changes. The change sets off a series of complex chemical internal reactions and feedback loops designed to restore balance. We have to respect this process and give our organisms time to adjusts to the initial shock of the stress stimulus, the damage itself, the organism's initial protective response to the damage, and the recovery from that response. Sometimes the recovery can take seconds like when we sneeze passing a flowering tree, sometimes hours, for example throwing up a bad batch of seafood a few hours after eating, sometimes weeks, for example when we fight off a head cold or virus, and sometimes months- the recovery of a broken limb or heart. We need to respect the healing process and give it the time it needs if we truly want to heal.

Little ones and healthy children and teens can often bounce back quickly but often they need time to recover too. It's important that they understand that the body needs to be heard and respected. Listening to the body is a skill which will serve them well into their adult life.

Tuning into the Body

Like tuning into a radio frequency, we have to learn how to focus on the body's needs and exclude the noise which surrounds us. I encourage parents to train their children to check in with their body. The body holds great wisdom. It knows what it needs. We just have to remind ourselves of that fact. When your child comes to the kitchen asking for a snack, or when they say they are hungry, ask them a few defining questions. Are you looking for something sweet or salty? Do you want something warm or something cool? Do you want something crunchy or creamy?

Sometimes kids head to the fridge or pantry when they are actually thirsty. Ask them to check in with themselves. Perhaps a juicy piece of fruit will fulfil their need for sweet and fluids, but sometimes they just need a glass of water.

You can also encourage them to check in with their body by asking if they are tired and need to lie down, or if they are feeing stagnant and need to move? Does the body need a hug, does it need a massage, maybe it needs to soak in a warm salt filed bath, maybe it needs lavender oil rubbed into the temples or calves, or a foot detox patch? Perhaps it needs to be in a quiet dark room, or to lie on the grass in the sun. This is an excellent exercise, especially for young children. Eventually they will be able to identify their specific needs and this will be of great help to you. Not just because it will make feeding them or managing their needs easier but because you'll start to see how these leanings point towards certain remedies. Remind them often that their body knows what it needs. And yes, sometimes it really does need chocolate ice-cream ;)

Potencies and Doses

One of the hardest things to understand when getting started with homeopathy is the different approach to dosing. We are used to taking medication for the duration of the disease and that makes sense when the purpose of the medication is suppressive rather than curative. But Homeopathy is founded on a different idea. The remedy is used to stimulate a vital molecular action and then if the action is strong enough, we allow the organism's own vital force and immune response to take over.

There are three homeopathic potency scales.

1. Centesimal Scale: 1:100 dilution ratio with 10 successions between each dilution- 12c, 30c, 200c (M- 1,000 x dilution) 1m, 10m, 50m
2. Decimal Scale: 1:10 dilution ratio with 10 successions between each dilution- 3x, 6x, 12x
3. Fifty millesimal Scale: 1:50,000 dilution ratio with 100 successions between each dilution - LM 6, 8, 10, 12, 14, 16, 18, 20 etc. or Q

Parents are best advised to stick to low potencies in the Decimal scale of
3x, 6x, 12x and Centesimal scale of- 30c and 200c. Sometimes c is also marked Ch.

I advise parents to start with a 30c for most ailments but there are some exceptions. High, fast-onset fevers and severe vomiting and/or diarrhea which don't respond to a 30c after an acute water dose (4 water doses over 1 hour) can be treated with a 200C.

If you see no change after the second or third water dose of a 30c, move on to a 200C. But if you see even the slightest change, wait. The organism needs time to reorganize itself.

Some people are very sensitive, and they respond better to one potency over another. It is highly individualized, and a certain amount of experimentation is required to get the correct potency match.

Often the aggravation from a higher potency can be quite strong so when treating the weak, the very young or elderly, always start slow and dose low.

GENERAL DOSING INSTRUCTIONS

VERY IMPORTANT- 1 dose means just that. Not once a day, not once a week, just once. One pill, or one sip, once.

1. Each time you take a dose, bang the closed bottle against the heel of the palm of your other hand or against a heavy book x10. This increases the potency slightly, so you are always increasing the stimulation.
 In Homeopathic dosing, the number 10 is important, do not add or subtract.
 2. Pop 1-2 pills into the lid, without touching and then directly under the tongue till dissolved or in water as advised. This is considered 1 dose.

WATER DOSE

When instructed, and for small children and infants, dilute 1 or 2 pills (or a quarter of a lid full of the poppyseed size pills), into a small amount of filtered or bottled (spring) water. Stir with a clean wooden stick or metal spoon till dissolved. Give approximately 5ml via a syringe, on a teaspoon, or in a sip. This is considered 1 dose.

WATER DOSE for ACUTES or EMERGENCY

 Dilute 1 or 2 pills in 1/4 small glass of filtered or bottled (spring) water. Take 5ml every fifteen minutes over 1 hour- a total of 4 doses, and then wait. If symptoms remain after a few hours, you can repeat. STOP dosing at any time if you see a change for better or worse. Things may get worse before they get better. This is an AGGRAVATION and it's a good sign that the remedy is acting.

 I suggest two pills just to be safe but if you have limited stock you may use one.

LM DOSING

Drop 2-3 drops of the LM liquid into a clean bottle of filtered or spring water. Bang the bottle x10 (or as advised), each time you take an approximate 5ml sip from the bottle. (Take as instructed- usually for 7-21days)

PLUSSING

Add 3 pills to 10 teaspoons of spring water. Take as directed leaving one spoonful in the bottle. Top up with an additional ten teaspoons and take as instructed by your homeopath.

CONSTITUTIONAL

Constitutional dosing should be as per instructions from your homeopath.

STORAGE & WHEN TO TAKE YOUR REMEDY

Take remedies 15 minutes away from food. No caffeine, mint or cannabis during the months following treatment please, or you will find yourself back where you started with a confused remedy picture.

Store remedies away from strong odors such as menthol, camphor, strong perfumes and essential oils, away from direct sunlight and **mobile and electronic devices.** These can and do interfere with remedies. If you need to keep them in your bag, or for transport, please wrap in aluminum foil and store in a pouch away from your mobile.

CHAPTER 7

Remedies for Home Treatment

As you become more familiar with homeopathy you will naturally want to treat your own family without calling your homeopath for every little accident, bite, rash or sting. I recommend you invest in a home remedy kit. If you're in England, I suggest the Helios kits because they are well packaged and easy to transport. There is also Hahnemann Labs and Washington Homeopathic Products, in the United States, amongst other. Find a supplier close to home and you will be well on your way.

The following remedy descriptions provide a very brief description of the action of the remedies and symptom pictures. I have tried to remain focused on family treatments for acutes, but some remedies lend themselves more to mental or emotional pictures. This doesn't mean you need the full emotional picture but if you do, it probably indicates a good choice. For example, you can confidently treat a hot, swollen bee sting with Apis. But if you have a child who is also a busy bee, clumsy and weepy, the remedy is sure to act well, not just locally, but constitutionally too.

Materia Medica is the **list of remedies** and their symptoms.
Repertory is a **list of symptoms** and their remedies.

You can search online for more detailed remedy descriptions. I highly recommend the Materia Media of the International Academy of Classical Homeopathy, which gives you access to the works of Kent, Boericke, Allan, Dunham, Farrington and Nash. For those looking for more on constitutional pictures, I recommend Essence of Materia Medica, by Vithoulkas and, The Soul of Remedies, by Rajan Sankaran.

< means worse from…

>means better from…

<u>Aconite</u>

Influenza, fever, conjunctivitis, ear infections, congestion, barking dry cough, shock and panic attacks. Sudden onset of any symptoms.

Aconite is like a great storm; it comes and sweeps over and passes away. -Kent

State of shock. **Panic attack**, fright, fear.

Ear problems after being out in the cold.

Sudden onset of any symptoms following exposure to cold wind, or cold bathing.

Burning hot head with cold body. Dry mouth, flushed face.

One cheek red, the other pale.

Vomits from fear.

Fear of death, fear of darkness, fear of bed, fear of ghosts. The patient looks like they have seen death.

Very thirsty for cold water.

Restless, palpitations, drowsy days, disturbed nights.

Retention of urine in infants following birth.

I have prescribed Aconite for patients who have panic attacks, when flying, when confined, or from general anxiety. It helps get through the state of panic. I also suggest parents keep Rescue Remedy on hand if they have panicky kids, or if they themselves tend to panic. People dealing with addiction withdrawal, or PTSD can take aconite as a temporary measure during the attack but should seek the help of a trained homeopath to treat the cause of the disturbance.

<cold, dry weather and cold winds, injury, surgery, shock

>sitting, walking, perspiration, open air

Desires: cold water

Ant-tart

Wet cough, bronchitis, vomiting from coughing, nausea.

Invaluable in diseases of the chest where the cough is provoked whenever the child gets angry, which is very often. - Farrington

Great accumulation of mucus in the lower respiratory tract, with no ability (or strength) to cough it up. **Rattling mucus and wheezing.**

Violent lower back pain.

Drowsy, cranky.

Irritable children with **aversion to being touched** or looked at. Children who don't want to be left alone.

Thirsty for cold water.

<In the evening, from lying down, in damp cold weather, warmth, from sour foods and milk.

> From sitting up, coughing up mucus, expelling gas and burping.

Desires: cold water and fruit, sour fruits, citrus fruits and apples

Apis

Stings, insect bites, oedema (fluid retention), allergies, inflammation, swelling.

*The skin symptoms and the patient are **aggravated from heat**. The face is greatly swollen at times, the **eyelids look like water bags**, the uvula* hangs down like a water bag...the mucus membranes look as if they would discharge water if punctured. - Kent*

*The uvula hangs down in the back of the throat between the tonsils.

Apis was first introduced into homeopathy after a severely oedemas (swollen) kidney patient was cured by dried honeybee powder prescribed by an indigenous medicine woman, in the mid 1800's.

Stinging, burning rashes and eruptions. When the sting creates **inflammation**, which is **red and hot** and pains which **sting and burn like fire** with **tremendous swelling**.
Puffiness under the eyes.
Suffocative feeling.
Hands and feet feel swollen, numb, puffed up.
Burning, stinging pains aggravated by heat.
Thirstless.
Apis can also be used for mild urinary tract infections with burning pains. It has an affiliation with the kidney.

Emotional and Mental Picture
A patient needing Apis can be awkward and clumsy, **dropping things easily**. They can be **jealous** and suspicious, with a **sharp tongue**, using words that sting. Often, they are industrious and like to work (**busy bee's**).
They can be very sensitive to constriction of any kind and can have a weepy disposition.

<Heat, during the night, after sleep.
>Cold applications, open air, sitting up, walking around.

Argentum Nitricum
Apprehension, performance anxiety, impulsivity, conjunctivitis, gastric complaints, nervous stomach.

Disturbance in memory, disturbance in reason. The patient is irrational, does strange things and comes to strange conclusions.- Kent

Open, **impulsive**, communicative and social, warm blooded, **aggravated by heat**.

Apprehension is felt in the stomach, butterflies in the stomach before a performance, event or even an appointment which makes him run to the toilet.

Belching with most **gastric complaints**, abdominal colic.

Ulceration of the stomach with radiating pain, chopped spinach stool, **fluids go straight through**.

Ulceration of the mucus membranes

Sharp, **splinter like pains** on swallowing, thick mucus.

Sleep is disturbed, sleepless from fancies of the imagination, bad dreams.

Overwhelming desire for sugar.

Emotional and Mental Picture

Nervous and fearful.

Impulsive

Hurried, restless, claustrophobic, panicky and **punctual.**

A young boy I treated once was a talented and funny actor and was often chosen for lead roles in his school plays. However, he suffered terribly from performance anxiety every time he had to go on stage, even though he enjoyed performing. He also had the strangest habit of feeling compelled to do anything he was warned against doing, including sticking his fingers in an automatic (electronic) device which was dangerous with a big warning not to touch! He had a great love of sweets, which were not good for him, was easily overheated, with a sensitive stomach and a poor short-term memory. A few doses of the remedy helped him with his performance anxiety and gave some much needed distance between the desire to act on impulse and the action of for example, opening the car door while in motion, another of his impulsive actions.

<warmth, at night, from cols foods, sweets, after eating, from emotions.

>fresh air, cold, pressure, burping.

Desires: sweets, sugar, salt.

Aggravated: Heat, (sweets which he desires) and excitement.

Arsenicum

Gastric conditions, diarrhea, vomiting, influenza, burning eyes, hay fever.

The essential process underlying Arsenicum is a deep-seated insecurity. The insecurity is not a lack of confidence on a social or professional level, but rather a more fundamental sense of vulnerability and defenselessness relating to disease and death. - Vithoulkas

Anxiety, **restlessness**, prostration (exhaustion), **burning pains** and deathly odors.
The chilly patient can't get warm.
Influenza and respiratory illness with burning pains. Hay fever with much sneezing, **burning** of eyes and **acrid** (burning, acidic) **runny nose** which burns the skin underneath.
Earaches better from warmth, worse from cold.
Burning pains in the chest,
Bad effects from eating too much fruit, **diarrhea, vomiting from food poison**. Cannot tolerate the smell of food.
Offensive discharges.
Very **thirsty for small sips** of water, wants warm drinks,
Anxiety, **fear of death, fear of being left alone.**
Great exhaustion after slight exertion.
Pale, cold, clammy, sweaty.
Tip of tongue red.
Worse midnight till 2am

Emotional and Mental Picture

Arsenicum is one of the most anxious remedies. They are chilly, anxious and restless. The patient, covered in blankets, moves from the sofa to the bed, from the bed to the kitchen, following the parent around the house. They don't want to be left alone, for fear they may die. They are pedantic and fastidious, **creating order** makes them feel safe in a world in which they feel threatened. They like to hold on to their material possessions collecting things they may need one day. There is a deep insecurity which can make their desire for order pathological.

I once treated an Arsenicum patient who hung his sox in pairs so they wouldn't get lost, which I thought was rather a good idea. But if he lost a sock in the wash or couldn't find the matching one, he could think of nor do anything else, until the missing sock was found. This is more than having an organized mind, this is pathology.

<cold, becoming cold, cold applications, worse at night, wet weather.
>Warmth, warm drinks, keeping the head up.

Belladonna
Sudden high fever state, ear infections (otitis), tonsilitis, headache from cerebral inflammation, mastitis.

Great intensity with sudden manifestation of symptoms. - Vithoulkas

Sudden, red, hot, throbbing picture. The face is flushed, the **cheeks are red**, **hot,** and dry, the **fever is high**, the ears are **throbbing.**
Bursting pains, red hot tonsils, the head hurts too much to move, every movement jars.
Pupils are dilated, the patient looks wild.
He doesn't want to be touched, very sensitive to light, to noise, everything aggravates.
Fever state. The child can get very cross.
Violence of symptoms, profuse urination, acuteness of all senses.
The skin is dry and hot to touch.
Sharp pains come and go.
No thirst with fever or can be very thirsty.
Grinding of teeth,
Restless sleep, the child startles when drifting off to sleep.
The hands or feet are ice cold, the face is burning hot.

< in the afternoon, after 3pm, and after midnight, from noise, touch, jar, draft. Worse from being uncovered.
>Being covered, resting in a quiet dark room undisturbed.
Desires - lemon or lemon juice

Bryonia

Colds and flu, bronchitis, burning congestion, fever, headaches, violent cough, sneezing, upper respiratory symptoms.

Bryonia patients are very sensitive to any intrusions; they are quick to feel irritability, anger or resentment. - Vithoulkas

The Bryonia patient is **irritable** and wants to be left alone. Even the **slightest movement aggravates**.

Slow onset of inflammation, often after exposure to cold winds, change of weather or emotional upset.

Fever without chills, with occipital headache (lower back of head), nausea and vomiting.

The **mucus membranes are dry** - the mouth, the tongue, the lips, the cough, the stool (constipation) are all dry. Loss of smell. Nosebleeds.

Pains are tearing and stitching, **all worse from movement**.

They are **very thirsty for large amounts** of water.

Dry, hacking cough forces them to sit up. The chest is so painful, the patient holds it when he coughs.

Unsatisfied, apprehensive, anxious, besotted, stupefied and dull.

Worse from eating, doesn't know what he wants.

Poor digestion, nausea, in stomach complaints relieved by warm drinks.

< motion, heat, eating.

>Rest, pressure (firm touch), cold.

Desires: warm milk

Calc-carb

Middle ear infections, enlarged glands, repeated swollen tonsils, gall stone colic, gastritis, tonsilitis, flu, respiratory conditions, mastitis, ulceration of nipple, poor milk.

Diseases arising from imperfect assimilation, imperfect ossification (bone formation), difficulty in learning to walk or stand. -Allan

The patient is tame, **chilly,** with **cold, clammy feet and tires easily. The metabolism is sluggish. Perspires easily, mostly at the back of the head.**
Babies **sweat profusely during sleep.**
Cal-carb children are fair, fat and flabby with a **sweet and stubborn disposition.**
During cold or fever state there is **weakness, heavy head,** eyes and limbs, with **lots of mucus from the nose** which blocks breathing.
Glandular affinity. Repeated glandular inflammation.
The tonsils are swollen, the uvula is red.
 Stitching pains extend to the ears, aggravated by swallowing, ameliorated by warm drinks.
Cough is dry in the morning, loose in the evening, worse from cold drafts, cold in general.
Diarrhea during teething, **difficult and delayed dentition, sour smelling diarrhea.**
Mastitis, aggravated by touch, ulceration of nipples, toothache or headache from nursing.
Night sweats.
Slow, sluggish metabolism, tendency to constipations.

Emotional and Mental Picture

As toddlers they are generally easy going and co-operative as long as they can do what they want in their own time. However, if you disturb them before they are ready - for instance if you need to pick up an older child from school and they have not finished the jigsaw - they can dig their heels in and make a big fuss. -Tricia Allan

Emotionally **Calc-carb children** are both **confident** and **reserved.** They like to check things out before committing. They can be **independent and stubborn,** as can Sulphur children but Calc-carb are not as self-centered. A better word to describe them might be **self-contained.** They don't like to be rushed. They need time to integrate and are often the last to leave the house. While they are intellectually bright, there is a slowness to their ability to process. **They need time**. This can make them appear indecisive. Once they have integrated or warmed up to an idea, and they get moving, they are bright, committed and hard working. Often the Calc-carb child will stay at the back of the class observing before joining in. But once they do, they are socially confident and take their place in the group often making some lifelong friends. They can **be late developers** and may have **many fears** including the dark, dogs, rats and insects and heights.

As adult they may fear for their children and fear losing their minds. They are sensitive to hearing cruel stories and are conscientious, hard-working and responsible.

< cold, wet weather, cold draft

>warmth, warm applications

*Desires: **eggs** (soft boiled), milky sweets, puddings, desserts, salt, child eats strange things.*

Aversion: milk

Calendula

Open cuts, wounds, slow to heal. Excessive pain disproportionate to the injury, eye injuries with pussy discharge. Lacerated scalp wounds.

Locally. For all wounds, the greatest healing agent. - Boericke

Injury to **muscles** and **tendons**.

Excessive bleeding after **tooth extraction**.

Chill with ailments, catch cold easily, especially in damp weather.

Sensitive to touch.

Post labor, caesarean.

<damp weather, heavy clouds, moving the sore part

>rest

Cantharis

Burns and raw burning pains. UTI's and bladder irritation, oversensitivity of all parts. Retained placenta with painful urination. Sunburn.

This is an intense remedy, the idea is that of fire, especially in the genitourinary system. ***Rapid, intense*** *and* ***destructive*** *symptoms. - Vithoulkas*

Burns, scalds, with **rawness** and smarting, relieved by cold.

Constant urge to urinate.

Rapid inflammation with great excitement and rage.

Cutting, **burning pains**.

Burning of soles of feet at night.

Very thirsty.

<touch, motion, pressure
>cold applications

I have used Cantharis to treat a throat that was burned by swallowing a piece of hot potato too quickly. Weeks later the patient was still aware of the area in her esophagus which had been burned. One dose of Cantharis in a low potency (30c) cleared it completely.

It is excellent for the first sunburn of summer when the children overdo it and turn lobster red.

Carbo-veg

Stagnation, low vitality, sepsis, easy fainting, collapsed.

The person feels that life is leaving him. - Vithoulkas

When emergency resuscitation is called for.

Debilitated, **must have air**, very weak, cold, **lifeless,** blue lips, cold from lack of blood circulation.

Nosebleeds, daily with pale face.

No energy in the muscles.

MUST be fanned, wants cold air.

Poor circulation and **imperfect oxygenation**. From loss of vital fluids, **from ill effects of exhausting disease. Faintness with cold perspiration.**

Pneumonia, breathlessness, great loss of blood.

<warm wet weather, rich foods, butter, fat.
>Open air, lying down, loosening tight clothes.

Chamomilla
Teething pains, colic, ear pains, uterine pains, toothache.

Loss of generosity; she has no consideration for the feeling of others. The awful pains that she is having, drive her to frenzy. This over sensitiveness to pain drives her to a mental state where she is unable to control her temper. -Kent

Oversensitive and irritable. Reactive. The nervous system is over excited. The child is in great pain and does **not want to be touched or spoken to**. Babies who are teething who **want to be carried all the time**. When they reach out for a toy and you give it to them, they throw it away, **capricious- nothing pleases them**, nothing distracts them from their discomfort. Ailments from anger.

One cheek is red (on the side where the tooth is breaking through), the other is pale.
Ringing in the ears, child **grabs at their ear in pain**, sharp shooting pains in ear.
Sensitive to smells, loss of smell with cold, runny nose makes it impossible to sleep.
Toothache from warm drinks or food.
Babies so miserable they **throw their head backwards, arching the back.**
Stool green and slimy with sore anus.

Unable to control their temper, **never satisfied**, doesn't know what she wants, goes from mother to the father.

Thirsty, hot, restless, snappish.

Pain in uterus.

<heat, anger, night, open air, wind.
>Being carried, rocked, warm damp weather.

China

Periodic fever, headaches, gall bladder and kidney pain, debilitating flue, snoring in children.

This is a touchy person. The nervous system is in a state of aggravation. Touch aggravates them in the physical and emotional level. - Vithoulkas

Seldom indicated in early stages of acute disease.

Debility from loss of vital fluid.

Liver, gallstone colic and spleen remedy.

Violent dry sneezing with inflammation.

Pains in limbs and joins, as if sprained, **worse from touch.**

Tearing, cutting pains.

Anemia, debility from disease, **post viral fatigue.**

Recurrent low-grade fever (same time every day or every second day etc.).

Tendency to congestion and inflammation.

Weak circulation with fullness of veins.

Chilly, sensitive to drafts, sensitive to touch.

<touch, pressure, drafts
>deep pressure (headaches)

Drosera

Dry cough, whooping cough, vomiting from cough, violent cough. Measles, Whooping cough.

Many complaints come on in the night, anxiety, sleeplessness and fear of ghosts. Fear of being alone. -Kent

Tickling, dry, **suffocative cough**. Vomits from coughing. **Spasmodic**, dry, irritating cough
Dusty feeling in throat makes him want to cough.
Yellow phlegm from cough or nose, nosebleeds.
Deep hoarse voice, laryngitis.
Loss of voice from speaking or singing- overuse.
Constriction of the throat preventing swallowing, **tickling from accumulated mucus in the larynx** causing **violent coughing** fits.
Often indicated in **Measles** and **Whooping cough.**
Pain between shoulder blades from coughing.
Bruised feeling from coughing, **patient must hold his chest**.
Fever with chill.

<lying down, eating and drinking, talking, becoming warm, after midnight.
>walking around, moving, open air, cool.

Gelsemium

Performance anxiety, muscular weakness, early inflammatory stage of colds and flu, collapsed feeling, weakness, debility. Measles.

Bad effects from fright, fear, exciting news and sudden emotion. -Allan

That shaky feeling you get from a cold or the flu, when you feel you must lie down, and you can barely keep your eyes open they are so heavy, the muscles feel so weak. That's the time to take a dose of Gelsemium.

Upper respiratory illness, **nasal congestion,** much sneezing with headache and fever.
Beginning stage of cold.

Shivers down the spine.

Dizziness, **heavy eyelids,** flushed face, hot.

The arms and legs feel heavy, tired, shaky.

The **muscles** feel paralyzed, **hard to move.**

Weakness and trembling.

Ailments from fright or **performance anxiety** bring on diarrhea. The child has to run to the toilet the **stomach is in a such state of nerves.**

< fright, excitement, emotional excitement, nerves.

>open air, movement, urination.

Hepar Sulph

Inflammation, infections, splinter like pains, ulcers, hay-fever, cold sores, infected pimples. Croup, loose rattling cough, hoarseness with loss of voice.

Oversensitive, physically and mentally. The slightest cause irritates him, quick, hasty speech and hasty drinking. - Allan

Localized inflammation with **pussy discharges.**

Very **sensitive to cold air,** it irritates the cough which starts up immediately after exposure.

Inflammation of **glands and tonsils with discharge,** which can **smell like rotten cheese.**

Throat **pain feels sharp, like a razor.**

Tendency to nasal discharge. Sinusitis with **thick offensive discharge.**

Chocking, gagging, croupy cough.

Tearing, bursting pains in ear with **thick, infected (smelly, yellow) discharge.**

Hyper-sensitive to all impressions.

Copious vaginal discharge with strong smell.

Oversensitive to pain, irritable and quarrelsome.

Destructive impulses.

Fear of bees and **stinging insects and needles.**

Easily offended, feels persecuted.

Concerned with appearances, feels unappreciated, **desires to kill, or to set on fire.**

<cold, exposure to draft, change in temperature, being uncovered.

>damp weather, warmth, warm drinks, warm wrapping.

Desire: fat and highly seasoned foods.

Hypericum
Injury to nerve rich parts - jammed fingers and toes, sore teeth.

Puncture injuries from nails or splinters. A hammer injury to **fingertips or the thumb.**

Jamming a toe or nail in a door.

Stitching, darting pains from the seat of the injury along the nerves.

Nails, spine, dental nerves.

Bruised coccyx following labor or a fall.

Headache extending to cheek bone.

Bunions and corns.

Lacerated fingertips, tongue. Gum pain following tooth extraction.

Hemorrhoids.

<touch, becoming cold.

Desires: warm drinks

Ignatia
Heartbreak, grief from unrequited love, moodiness, sighing.

Absorbed in grief - Guernsey

This is a wonderful remedy for teens or tweens who are pining after a loved one. The grief is so deep, she cries in her room alone, and even when she comes out to join the family, she can't hide her pain. Many thoughts.

Grief from **loss of a loved one**.

Divorce, separation, rejection.

Aversion to consolation, **heavy sighing**, can't quite catch her breath.

Lump in the throat with grief.

Changeable mood. Silent brooding, sighing and **sobbing**.

Sinking feeling in stomach, relieved by deep breath.

Prolapse, stitching pains in rectum, stools pass with difficulty.

Sensitive souls, often creative, artistic, refined with a tendency to hysteria because she is so sensitive.

Aversion to tobacco smoke, **aversion to fruit**.

Spasms in children from fright.

<in the morning, open air, after a meal, coffee, smoking.
>While eating.

Ipecacuanha

Nausea, excessive salivation, nausea with any complaints; fever, gastric complaints, vomiting while coughing.

Ipecacuanha leads all the remedies for nausea.

All complaints are **accompanied by extreme nausea**.

Blocked up nose with nausea, headache with nausea, menstruation with nausea.

Constant nausea with much salivation.

Green stool with colic and nausea.

Ailments from anger, vexation.

<veal, lying down, humid wind

Kali-bichromium

Stringy, ropey discharge. Thick mucus discharge, from eyes, nose, ears, vagina.
Postnasal drip, rattling respiration difficult expectoration. Sinusitis.

In this remedy, stickiness is the main idea. The mind, the emotions, the discharges, are stuck. Sticky thoughts, sticky puss, sticky discharges, sticky vomiting. The pains do not move, they are stuck in a spot. -Vithoulkas

Effects the **mucous membranes** and air passages.
Thick and copious nasal discharge, green, yellow.
Sinus headaches- over eyebrows, with **thick nasal congestion**.
Pressure and **pain at root of nose. Loss of smell, violent sneezing**.
Sore bones of the face.
Chronic weeping of the **middle ear**- secretion more mucus than puss.
Discharge **yellow, thick, sticky**, with stitching pains (predominantly left ear).
Hacking cough, brings up **thick sticky mucus**. Violent cough with wheezing.
Ropey vomiting.
Thick and jelly like vaginal discharge- leucorrhea.
Duodenal ulcers.
Pain in finger-tip sized spots.

<beer, summer heat, 2-3am
>heat, pressure
Desires: sweets, beer
Aversion: water, meat

Kali-carb
Irritability, oversensitivity to pain, anxiety felt in the stomach- solar plexus. Bloated stomach, gassy, stuffed up nose, throat pains, dry cough. Rigid type.

Overuse of the mind as a mechanism for control. There are many remedies for the complaints of kali-carb but look for the type. The child or partner who is inflexible in his or her ways, controlled, rigid, duty bound and irritable and where the anxiety is expressed in the solar plexus. -Vithoulkas

Nose stuffed up in warm room, sticking pain in throat, violent cough.

Small baglike **swelling - upper** and lower **lids**.

Very **sensitive to drafts**.

Aversion touch, fearful.

Sharp cutting pains.

Hypersensitive to pain.

Distended stomach, immediately after eating. Everything turns to gas. Pain in right hypochondria (upper abdomen). Flatulence, constipation, diarrhea - 2am-4am.

Soles of feet very sensitive.

Backache, sciatica, lumbago - better by walking, gets up in the middle of the night to walk. Can't turn over in bed.

Unrefreshed sleep, worse 2-5am.

Emotional and Mental Picture

Dogmatic, inflexible, proper, upright, over mentalization. Anxiety felt in the stomach. Sensitive, easily frightened.

Sensitive to environmental changes and emotions yet they don't share or show their emotions. Can be **irritable**. Inability to cope with loss of control.

<In cold weather, coffee, soup, lying on painful side (left), 2-5am

>moving around, daytime, doubling over - pressure.

Desire: sweets

Lachesis

Swelling and inflammation of the throat. Circulation issues - hot flushes. High blood pressure. Feelings of constriction. Left sided aggravations - moving to right.

Great sensitivity of and around the throat, **cannot bear constriction** of any kind such as tight clothes or a scarf. Suffocative feeling.

Difficulty swallowing, sore throat, better swallowing solids. Tonsils better from cold drinks, worse from hot.

Lump in throat with **constant desire to swallow**.

Earache with sore throat.

Hay-fever with much sneezing during the day, wakes into attack.

Bronchitis, pneumonia, **left side**. Suffocative cough, worse on going to sleep.

Dry tongue.

Dark, purple, **mottled, discoloration** on the skin - ulcers, skin eruptions, tonsils.

Headaches from the sun.

Sleeps into headaches, wakes feeling bad.

Painful stool, offensive, anus feels closed.

Asthma cough during sleep, cough excited by touch on the throat.

Gastric disturbances - **cannot tolerate anything tight** around the abdomen.

Mastitis with blue or red discoloration of mammae. Cystitis from retention.

Ailments from **jealousy** and **suppressed expression**.

Loquacious - talkative. Suspicious, jealous, self-loving, impulsive, insanity.

< sleep, spring, pressure, constriction, left side, closing eyes,

>discharge, warm applications, pressure, cold.

Ledum

Stings and bites, wounds, gout, tetanus.

Injury from stepping on tacs, from puncturing with needles, wounds that bleed scantily but are followed by pain, puffiness or coldness of the part. -Kent

I have found ledum tincture to be very useful topically on mosquito bites in those who are sensitive, especially in tropical climates.

Stings and **bites** with **hard swellings, cold to touch.**

Ulcers **better with cold applications**, penetrating **wound injuries**.

Tetanus where the injured part is cold.

Rheumatic pains, right hip or left shoulder. Gout, cellulitis, sprains.

All injuries better from very cold applications.

<warmth, and movement

\>cold application, cold water (bathing)

Lycopodium

Bloating, gastric complaints, urinary and digestive disturbances, styes, head colds with nasal discharge, earaches with discharge.

nervous excitement and prostration are marked. -Kent

Head colds with discharge from the nose- thick, copious, yellow.

Nasal passage obstructed (in babies, causing mouth breathing).

Discharge from ears, offensive.

Acute sense of smell.

Tickling cough.

Headaches which are better with open air, cool, worse from being warm, though the patient himself is cold and wants to be warm. Periodical headaches.

Prefers warm drinks for the sore throat, warm meals, and warm applications in general.

Cramps in calves and toes at night, twitching and jerking of limbs on falling asleep, pain in heels.

Burning between scapulae.

Ravenous hunger but fills ups fast. Eating increase the appetite. But eating produces gas which causes **bloating**, pain and a feeling of fullness. Flatulence, gas, right sided remedy.

Must eat regularly or he will get a headache.

Constipation with ineffectual urging.

Sensitive to cold, **lack of vital heat.**

Very sensitive, oversensitive to pain.

With pains caused by **inflammatory conditions**, such as Rheumatoid arthritis or fever, he is **relieved by the warmth of the bed**, but he is also **restless, tossing** and turning in pain all night.

Delirium with fever.

Flow of urine slow to get started.

Impotence in men.

Kidney colic.

Emotional and Mental Picture

Likes to show off but inside he feels insecure and weak. -Vithoulkas

The little (and big) Lycopodium is **timid and cowardly** inside but when he feels safe around those weaker than himself, he becomes **dictatorial**. **Fears** ghosts, **being alone in the house.** Does not want company but does not want to be alone either. His memory is weak, he **forgets words** and makes mistakes when writing. He **fears performing** in public or giving a presentation, even when he has done it many times, and fears commitment and taking on new responsibilities. Nervous, sensitive, emotional, cries when being thanked.
Distrustful, fault finding and suspicious. Gets angry easily.

All symptoms worse 4pm-8pm and on waking.
<4pm-8pm, heat, warm room, hot air
>movement, warm food and warm drinks, cooling down, being uncovered
Desires: warm food and drinks, sweets.

Mag-phos

Cramps, spasms, headaches, ear pain, stomach cramps, spasmodic cough- whooping cough, tooth ache, teething. Colic in babies. Writer's cramp, muscular weakness.

Acts on the nerves and muscles -Vithoulkas

Mag-phos is one of the **leading remedies for cramps.**
Muscle cramps, leg cramps, stomach cramps and **menstrual cramps** lend themselves well to being treated by Magnesium- phosphorous.
Gastric pains and cramps **better from bending or doubling over**, and better from warmth, a hot water bottle, heated rice pack, or a warm bath relieve.
Gas and burping do not bring relief.
Neuralgic head and **tooth pains**- better from heat and pressure.
Menstrual cramps, better with warmth.

Angina - constricting cardiac pains.

Teething in babies.

Usually, symptoms do not come with a fever but are of a muscular nature. The patient complains about her pain, **moaning** about the house. Think of a teenage girl moaning about menstrual cramps, lying on her bed **doubled over in pain**, with a hot water bottle to bring relief. She will be helped by this remedy.

< cold, touching the sore area, right side, night

>warmth, doubling over or sitting in pose of a child position, pressure, rubbing.

Mercurius - (Sol or Vive)

Offensive discharges, excessive salivation, metallic or salty taste, offensive breath, indented tongue, profuse perspiration, mild stammering, mouth sores, tonsilitis, otitis-ear infections, pneumonia, conjunctivitis, cystitis, offensive discharges. Sinusitis.

White coated **tongue, indented** with **teeth marks**, swollen.

Sore throat, tonsilitis, with **offensive breath** - infection.

Nasal **discharge, green**, excessive.

Pain in head on blowing the nose and stooping down.

Pneumonia, Bronchitis, worse lying on right side.

Bleeding gums, inflammation of gums, **mouth sores, ulcers**.

Worse with **extreme cold** or **extreme heat** - think of mercury's sensitivity to temperature.

Violent thirst, hiccups, salivation especially during sleep.

Emotional and Mental Picture

Rude, critical, suspicious, feels threatened. Weak memory, forgetful, talks fast, hurried.

<night, warmth of bed, heat, damp weather

>sleep, cold, sour food

Desires: bread and butter, cold drinks,

Natrum-muriaticum

Dry mucus membranes, weakness, head colds, nasal and upper respiratory congestion, headaches. Bed wetting. Craves salt. Dandruff. Herpes around the mouth- cold sores.

Nat-mur is a deep and long-acting remedy. It takes a wonderful hold of the economy (the organism), making changes that are long lasting when given on potentized (homeopathic) doses. -Kent

Head colds start with much **sneezing**. Violent nasal discharge, nasal obstructions, discharge like **raw egg white**.
Hammering headaches, pressing pain, worse from the heat of the sun.
Stomach- constipation unusually hard, chronic diarrhea.
Tendency to emaciate (lose weight) even while eating well.
Involuntary urination during activity or from coughing or sneezing.
Enuresis in children- **bed wetting.**
Very thirsty remedy.

Emotional and Mental Picture

Avoids being hurt at all costs. Fear of rejection, fear of ridicule. -Vithoulkas

Repeated **grief** leaves them feeling the need to self-protect. A child or teenager may close themselves up, shut down emotionally, become unreachable after being repeatedly shamed or ridiculed. It is a very **sensitive** remedy. For example, a constitutional Nat-mur will be modest about going to the toilet in public and when upset he wants to cry in private, consolation **(sympathy) aggravates**. It is an emotional remedy with a focus on rejection, shame and grief. He protects himself by closing up and becoming emotionally independent. Thinks about unfortunate things that happened, **goes over them in his mind**. Delicate children, sensitive to disharmony. Hysterical laughing/weeping. Depression. Periodicity- meaning he gets regular headaches or asthma attacks usually at the same time of day, or once a week etc. Fastidious, fear of germs. **Perfectionists**. Irritable

< heat of the sun, 10am-11am, cold

>open air, pressure against back.

Desires: salt

Aversion: fat of meat, slimy food.

Nux-vomica

Digestive complaints, ulcers, spasms, headaches and nausea from overindulgence. Sour vomiting. Nausea. Lockjaw. Lower backache. Hay fever, sinusitis. Toothache. Chilly.

Sudden and intense onset of symptoms.

Itching in the eustachian tube (ear) sneezing in the morning. Running nose with scraping sensation in throat. Nose runs during the day and is blocked at night.

Sore throat causes coughing.

Scraping feeling in larynx, violent cough in morning.

Cough brings on **bursting headache**. Cough better with warm drinks.

Better in open air, worse in a closed warm room.

Over-indulgence created **disorder in the digestive system.**

Fever with gastric complaints.

Nausea in morning after eating or indulging in stimulants.

Pressure in stomach after eating little. **Colic, gas.** Frequent **ineffectual desire** for stool and urination.

Nausea in morning during menstruation.

Sensitive to pain, smell, noise.

The **nervous system** is **sensitive**.

Pain after dental work.

Emotional and Mental Picture

Ambitious, intelligent, capable and competent with a strong work ethic. Self-reliant.

Overly ambitious and competitive. Fastidious with an emphasis of efficiency. **Fault finding**. Drawn towards stimulants, coffee, tobacco etc. to keep up with his drive to succeed. Does not tolerate contradiction. Can be malicious and cruel, impulsive and reactive. **Easily irritated**.

<cold dry weather, being cold, draft, uncovering, after eating, stimulants, 9am
>wet weather, a warm room, after passing stool, from an undisturbed rest.
Desires: spicey foods, rich foods, stimulants.

Phosphorus
Bleeding nose, easy bleeding, profuse menstruation, anxious, fast growth spurts, very thirsty for cold drinks. Burning pains, digestive complaints, nausea and vomiting. Loss of voice with laryngitis, cough from tickling in throat.

Diffusion is the theme which runs through the Phosphorus pathology. -Vithoulkas

Lanky teens who **grow too fast**, weak limbs, apathetic, talk slowly, low energy.
Irritation and **inflammation** the mucus membrane. Bleeding gums.
Raw inflamed tonsils, swollen, bleeding, with intense pain, inability to swallow, and **loss of voice.**
Bronchitis, Pneumonia, pain in chest, and between scapula, **heat running up the spine** and in spots between bones of the spine.
Congestive, **throbbing headaches**. Worse from movement and heat, better for cool applications or being in a cool room and from rest.
Burning brain. Violent head pains, with hunger. **Meningitis**, swelling of the brain, excess heat.
Violent neuralgia- nerve pain.
Hunger soon after eating. **Hungry at strange times**, must eat. Burning in esophagus.
Bloody discharges.
Sensitive to changes in weather and **electrical storms.**
Exhaustive conditions. General weakness, they must lie down.
Sensitive to all external impressions, sight, sound, noise, smell, touch.
Restless, fidgety.

Dandruff, **hair falls out**.

In fever state, chilly with cold hands and feet.

Stiffness on beginning to move, Rheumatic stiffness, drawing tearing pains.

<u>Emotional and Mental Picture</u>

Phosphorous children are delightful and full of enthusiasm for life. They are friendly and outgoing, love having people around them and have a magnetic personality. -Tricia Allan

Warm and **affectionate**, social. Can be naïve, trust easily and are easily magnetized. They are also attractive and popular as people are drawn to them because they are open, affectionate and **sympathetic**. They are daydreamers and thus easily startled as they are suddenly pulled back into themselves, for example at the sound of loud thunder during a storm. They can also be quite **anxious** and fearful, and they **prefer company**. **Fears** of dark, **being alone**, something happening to themselves or loved ones, loud noises. Sometimes the anxiety has no known source. Clairvoyance.

One Phosphorus child I treated for exhaustion, was always worried that her mother would run out of gas or miss a turn on the way to school, though neither of these things had ever happened. She was a lovely and easy-going child, very sympathetic, friendly, and open. Loved by her teachers and school friends. Socially independent and affectionate. Even though she was quite confident, she didn't like being left at home alone, even during the day, and preferred someone to be in the house, even though she didn't particularly need to engage with them. She also loved a good massage and was very thirsty for cold drinks. These keynotes confirmed the remedy, to which she responded well.

<exertion, touch, warm food, getting wet in hot weather, electric storms, oysters.
>In the dark, open air, cold bathing, sleep, being massaged.
Desires: ice-cream, cold foods, sweets, chocolates, fish, salty foods, cold drinks.

Pulsatilla
Nasal discharge, ear pain, loose cough, sinusitis, weepiness and clinginess, conjunctivitis, flue, cystitis, diarrhea, thirstless in all complaints.

All symptoms are aggravated from warmth of room or bed and ameliorated in open air, open windows, continued motion. - Vithoulkas

Symptoms change, **changeable picture**, emotionally and physically.

Throat painful, scratchy.

Thick **yellow mucus** streaming from the nose.

Discharge from ears, painful.

Headaches from working too hard.

Styes, Crack in middle of lip.

Bitter or salty taste.

Aversion to fats and rich foods.

The constitution is hot, they **must have air**, must be fanned, cooled down.

Teething babies present with **one red check**. (Chamomilla babies can also have one red cheek, but they are really cross about their pain, capricious.)

Emotional and Mental Picture

Children who need Pulsatilla are soft and gentle, and very sensitive to the big wide world they find themselves in. They are shy and timid, constantly seeking affection and reassurance from their parents and other adults. - Tricia Allan

Mild natured, timid, **cry easily**, **weepy** and **clingy**. Many fears, abandonment, separation. A new sibling can evoke jealousy which will make them even more demanding. Pulsatilla babies don't like to be put down. Older children don't like to sleep alone and will come to their parent's bed if they wake at night. Generally, these are the most sensitive of children, weepy, tearful, delicate, full of insecurities and fears.

<warmth, lying on back

>open air, cold applications

Aversion: fat, thirstless with all complaints

New babies and sibling rivalry

Sibling rivalry may be established from the first moment an older child sees their mother with a new baby in her arms. If the mother has not birthed at home and the older child has not been present during the birth, an older sibling coming into a new family dynamic (especially one from which they have already been excluded), can be emotionally confronting, and may establish an emotional pattern of rivalry. So the first time the older sibling see's the new baby, someone other than the mother should be holding her. A grandparent, neighbor, aunt, uncle or family friend can hold the newborn, so the child first sees their mother without the newborn in her arms. Then ask the child if they would like to hold **their** new baby. Sit the older child down near the mother, and hand the new, well swaddled and firmly supported bundle to the child to hold. Young children will hold the baby for a few minutes before handing it back to the mother. This allows the older child to feel safe, still loved (what a relief!) and somewhat responsible for the wellbeing and care of the new baby, instead of feeling threatened by his or her arrival.

Rhus-tox-

Hives, Poison Ivey, chicken pox, shingles, intensely itchy better from heat. Stiff muscles, sciatica, lumbago. All pains wore from rest, better from movement.

Affects the fibrous tissue - especially right side. - Allan

Musculoskeletal affections ameliorated by motion and warmth and aggravated by being still. -Vithoulkas

Restless, must move, cannot stay in one position too much time because of the pain.
Sore **muscles**, strained muscle or **tendon, stiffness**, fever with aching muscles.
Limbs **stiff and weak**, stiff knees, stiff neck, **lumbago**, cracking joints, all better from heat and movement. But too much movement causes fatigue.

Small of the back painful.

Rheumatic conditions, **pains in the bone**.

Rash, hives - very itchy, no relief. Skin red hot and burning, worse with exposure to cold air, better for warmth.

Chicken pox, itchy, **hives itch with no relief.**

Inflammation of eyes, **spasmodic sneezing, sore throat**, inflammation and **swelling of esophagus.**

Red tip of the tongue.

Thirsty with dry mouth and tongue.

Eczema of the scalp in infants.

Styes, lower lid. Discharge from the eyes.

Emotionally sad, restless, apprehensive, irritable, anxious.

<cold, wet rainy weather, rest, lying on back, getting up.

>warm, dry weather, movement, walking, change of position, stretching limbs, a warm bath

Desires cold milk or has aversion to it.

Ruta

Injuries to joints, tendons, ligaments, connective tissue. Bursitis, nodules following injury. Overstraining of eyes. Headaches from eye strain.

Sprains to wrists and ankles.

Bruised feeling in spine and limbs.

Can't get comfortable, restless, everything feels bruised and tender.

Shortening of tendons, contraction of **fingers, sciatica** from hip to thighs, worse bending.

Pain from **overstretching** or **injury to muscles and ligaments.**

Bone pains in feet and ankles.

Eye strain, **burning eyes** from being overly focused.

Constipation, straining, prolapse of rectum.

Paralysis of bladder from overextension.

Eruptions of skin with severe itching.

Weakness and tiredness.

Jaundice.

<lying down, cold, wet, 10am, walking up and down stairs

>Rubbing, walking, motion, pressure, lying on non-injured side.

Sepia

Hormonal complaints, exhausted mothers, morning-sickness, prolapse, constipation during pregnancy, hot flushes during menopause. Fever blisters, crack lower lip. Bedwetting.

Indifference to those whom she loves best. - Allan

The Sepia patient says, "I know I ought to love my children and my husband, I used to love them, but now I have no feeling on the subject." - Kent

Action on the **hormonal system**. The Sepia woman creates a protective shield around herself to give herself a much-needed emotional and physical break from the demands of motherhood. Sepia is made from the ink of the cuttlefish which ejects a, ink screen to get away from her predators.

Great **indifference**, she sits and stares, feels nothing, and then when demands are made, (as they always are on the new mother), she tries to meet them, but she is so **depleted** and empty. Sometimes she will lose control and scream at her family and children.

Desire to escape, but dread of being alone. Restless, frustrated, irritable, argumentative, broken down, **no enthusiasm**.

Hot flushes during menopause, weakness, sweating. **Night sweats**, sweat from least exertion.

Aversion to sex, no energy for it.

Hair falling out during menopause.

Constipation during pregnancy.
Prolapse of uterus and vagina. Bearing down sensation during menstruation. Pain travels down into the thighs. Bearing down pains.
Burning vaginal discharge before menstruation.
Pre-menstrual tension.
Bedwetting in children, during the first sleep, the action of the sphincter is weak.

Morning-sickness, headache in morning with nausea, **nausea** after eating, and nausea better from eating, aversion to smell of cooking, burning in pit of stomach.
Headache left temple, or pumping right sided, dizziness, nosebleeds. Chilly.
Emotionally Sepia can have a sharp tongue and a be sarcastic and seem callous. She is perceptive and detached.

<cold, sex, pregnancy, morning, cloudy weather, before thunderstorm, before periods, doing the laundry or domestic work, dampness.
>Dance, movement, exercise, warmth of bed, warm applications, food, after a sleep, pressured touch, afternoon.
Desires: sweets, alcohol, vinegar
Aversion: smell of cooking, meat, salt, fat, bread

Silicia

Cysts, hard warts, scoliosis. Performance anxiety. Blocked tear duct in babies. Sinusitis, ear infections, skin abscess, mastitis, cracked nipples, cutting pain during nursing, suppressed milk flow. Ingrown toenails.

Chilly, weak patients with **profuse perspiration** and a tendency to catch cold. **Lack of vital heat.** One of the **coldest of all the remedies** - wears a hat in bed.
Sinusitis with thick discharge, post-nasal drip.
Otitis - ear infections with thick discharge. **Chronic** swollen glands, inflamed with suppuration - discharge, puss.

Sweaty feet, acrid - **acidic**.

White spots on nails, warts.

Toothaches and sore gums.

Coccyx injuries - the bed feels too hard.

Inactive rectal muscle, **constipation**, stool is dry, recedes.

Promotes expulsion of foreign bodies - **produces inflammation and suppuration**.

Wounds heal slowly.

Mastitis, sore, bruised, hardening of breast tissue like stones, suppressed milk flow, aversion to mother's milk.

Emotional and Mental picture

Refined, sensitive, lacking in stamina, **delicate**. Timidity from lack of nervous resilience.

Fears performing or taking on a new project but pushes herself to meet the challenge and succeeds. **Timid** and **yielding** but **obstinate**. Silica can be fixed in her ideas, but she doesn't have the energy to argue too much.

Obstinate, headstrong children, cry when spoken kindly to. Fidgety, anxious, easily startled. **Nightwalking**.

<cold, change of weather, during menstruation, becoming cold and wet, effected by moon both new and full.

>Warmth, being wrapped up, head coverings, summer, resting.

Desires: warmth, eggs

Aversion: meat, salt, fat, warm foods.

Staphisagria

Anger, indignation, head pain, crumbling teeth, cystitis post-surgical wounds, eczema, styes on lids. Honeymoon cystitis. Sensitive. Eczema, fig warts.

The whole mind and nervous system are in a fret. -Kent

A remedy of **suppressed anger**. Suppressed emotions, usually felt about a partner.
Oversensitivity on all levels. Feels emotionally neglected, unappreciated.

Sensitive, sweet, **easily offended**, gentle people who suppress their anger, until it explodes in a violent outburst, but never violent enough to do real harm. Even in their anger, they are sweet.

Ailments from grief in the form of stomach aches, hair falling out, psoriasis, involuntary movements - effects of the nervous system.

The tips of the fingers are sensitive, sometimes numb with tingling sensation - crawling inside.

The ears are sensitive to loud noise, sensitive to smell, to taste.

Headaches from anger.

Dry sensitive warts around genitals, fleshy warts.

Extreme hunger after eating.

Cystitis from excess sex, **burning in urethra** when not urinating.

Post-surgery - cutting pains. **Tender scars** (physical and emotional).

Sensitive to reprimand but won't cry, instead they will internalize it.

<afternoon nap, wakes moody, unrefreshed. Anger, tobacco.

>warmth, rest, after eating in the morning.

Desires: Tobacco

Sulphur

Hot, dry, itching skin, burning pains, congested, flushes of heat. Tonsilitis, cystitis, fevers and flue, diarrhea offensive. Acidic. Burning feet at night, itching scalp.

Lean, lanky hungry, sedentary. The ragged philosopher, the scholar. - Herring

Burning pains better with cold applications, **red, hot** lips, anus, eyes, ears, especially during fever.

Conjunctivitis, **sandy** deposits in **eyes in morning**.

Offensive discharges from ears, itching inside and/or outside ear.

Offensive perspiration.

Constipation - **child afraid to pass stool** - painful, knotty, dry.

Morning diarrhea will drive them out of bed.

Offensive stool.

Very thirsty with a preference for cold drinks. Sweet, cold drinks, like apple juice.

Must eat by mid-morning, cannot wait to eat, feels faint from not eating.

Eczema - **dirty looking skin**, dry, hot, very itchy. **Worse from warmth of bed**, woolen clothing. Cannot wear wool.

Heat on **top of head** and **soles of feet**. Stick feet out of covers.

When the best selected remedy for worms fails.

Pain in prostate, painful ejaculation.

Bedwetting in grubby, (scrofulous - sickly) children.

Troubled sleep.

As adults even though they may present well, there is always some area that reveals this disorder, it can present on the skin, on a patch of eczema or in an offensive discharge. Some adults - usually men, who **do not care about their appearance. Standing for long periods is difficult**. You will find them slouched over an armchair or lazing on the couch.

Emotional and Mental Picture

Philosophical types, intelligent. Quick tempered, **critical**, selfish, anxious, **hurried.** Irritable, depressed, thin, weak, even though they eat well. No regard for the feelings of others. Fear heights, **worries about his children**, fear germs and contamination. Religious melancholy.

Fiercely independent children, grubby and unaware of the chaos they leave around them**, highly explorative**. Curious about how things work. They will pull something apart just to see how it works. Very **bright** children, **precocious**. The Sulphur child will talk to strangers easily and with confidence, but they are **not pleasers**. They will walk away or ignore you if they lose interest. (Sulphur adults can do the same). Children dressed like Pippi Long-stockings, they do not care that their clothes are on backwards or stained with blueberries. While they love to play in water, they do not like to have to wash, they **do not like to have to do anything**.

<warmth of bed, standing, washing, milk disagrees

>cold applications, cold drinks, lying down, resting, catnaps, massage

Desires: sweets, cold drinks, sweet cold drinks, fat, alcohol, well-seasoned foods

Aversion: Bathing, eggs (but if there is a strong Calc-carb underlying layer they may crave eggs). Sour foods, strong cheese.

CHAPTER 8

Natural Immunity

Our children are not Autistic, they are Autoxic.

In that cozy macro kitchen where I first learned about healing foods, I also came to understand some things about the invasive medical procedures we had come to accept without question, and their impact on our health; the excessive prescribing of antibiotics and pharmaceutical medications, routine surgeries, the dramatic increase in convenient C-sections and perhaps the most sinister and damaging of all, the mass vaccine programmes.

At the time, search engines were a little less user friendly than they are today, but I was able to source enough information, to alert my interest. My husband had graduated with a BSc. majoring in biochemistry, so he was able to read and understand published studies and explain them to me in lay terms. Many nights were spent deep in discussion about the impact of introduced chemicals on the natural and delicate biochemical exchanges. We understood enough to decide that we would defer vaccinating our children, until we were convinced otherwise.

The hostility we faced from family, doctors and nursing staff in the hospital in which our first child was born, was enough to raise some serious red flags. Surely, I had every right as a mother to research something as invasive as a vaccination before allowing it to be injected into my infant child? Why the hostility? Were the doctors and nurses more educated about the subject than I was, and if so, I was willing to hear them out? But their party line answers to my questions about vaccine safety, gave me cause to suspect they were not. I had graduated with a degree in visual communication, so I could spot a marketing campaign a mile away. The pamphlets they handed out and from which they quoted, were the things I myself was trained to design and write. I was not fooled by their glossy finish or their slick copy and I was surprised how many intelligent educated medical professionals were.

Our family doctor at the time was a gentle, kind and open-minded man. His community surgery in Bondi Beach, Sydney, had an influx of drug users he treated routinely with intravenous vitamin C protocols for hepatitis. He was open enough to admit that he too had researched vaccines for his children and he supported our decision not to vaccinate ours.

Ten days before the due date of our second child, our oldest came home from school with the chicken pox. In order to prevent the baby from catching it if I should go into labor, I was given an immunoglobulin, (antibodies against the disease), which set me off into early labor. The baby was protected, but ten days after a difficult home birth, I came down with a severe infection of the varicella zoster virus (chicken pox).

Apparently, I had not been exposed to the virus as a child, which left me nursing a ten-day old baby with a high fever and painful pox sprouting all over my body. It was a very difficult time, and I came to understand why it was so important to allow our children to catch these childhood diseases during childhood. I was happy that my daughter had been infected and would now carry lifelong immunity. The chicken pox vaccine was relatively new at the time, and while available, was not mandatory, yet.

Two years later, we were blessed to have the opportunity to spend some time in the magnificent rainforests of northern New South Whales, where the community was steeped in nature and alternative ideologies. We enrolled our oldest in a local Waldorf school where soon after there was a measles outbreak in the largely unvaccinated local population. Within a few weeks our daughter came out with classic upper respiratory symptoms, and a high fever, followed a few days later by the typical measles rash, and her younger sister followed suite.

It was one of the hottest summers on record, with bushfires spreading all the way along the coast. The land was scorched, and we were housebound. I rushed to hang make-shift curtains on the glass windows which looked out onto the forest, to protect their eyes from the light, and I sent my husband into town to stock up on vitamins and homeopathic and herbal remedies. I won't lie and say that it was easy to nurse two small children through the measles, but I had made a decision to be a mother, I had carried and birthed these children, I had it within me to see them through the Measles. This is how mothers are grown.

It was during this time that I realized how disempowered women have become. Our ancestors consulted their mothers, aunts and wise women of their tribes and villages, and we were emboldened by that ancient lineage which was grounded in traditional and powerful healing wisdom. But somewhere along the lines, that was broken and women became dependent on the medical and drug industry to heal their own children from even the most minor ailment. For me, it was important to work through the fear and step into my power as a woman and as a mother and reclaim my rightful inheritance as a healer and medicine woman for my own family.

When our third was born, again we declined vaccines. Our three little girls played freely with their vaccinated cousins and friends and they went to school without much fuss, but we were asked to keep them home during outbreaks which we happily did. When the department of health issued permission forms for school vaccinations, I marked ALLERGIC-NO PERMISSION across the whole page in a big black marker and kept them home just to be safe. To date, I can count the number of times my five children have collectively been on antibiotics on one hand and their childhood visits to the doctor and dentist, on two.

In 1986, US president Ronald Reagan signed The National Childhood Vaccine Injury Act, protecting vaccine manufacturers from litigation, leaving parents of vaccine damaged children completely unsupported, and left to pick up the pieces of their shattered lives alone. If anyone even suggested that vaccines were directly responsible for their children physical, emotional, behavioral and developmental decline and death they were ostracized and ridiculed by doctors and so-called experts.

By 1998, when the Pharma-funded, media persecution of Dr. Andrew Wakefield made its way across our television screens, I had done enough research to know that vaccines were a toxic assault on the immune system and a crime perpetrated against our children and against us mothers and parents. We were knowingly deceived, by the very well-oiled marketing divisions of corrupt vaccine manufacturers, into co-facilitating the injury of our own children. It doesn't get more evil than that.

Each and every parent of a vaccine damaged child says these haunting words, "my child was perfectly healthy until they were vaccinated". Any attempt to invalidate these parents is, in my opinion, a cowardly reaction of denial of a truth too difficult to face.

I am willing to concede that there are other contributing factors to the rise in chronic childhood illness. These include our toxic food systems, environmental toxins, fluoride in our water, chemicals sprayed onto our kitchen surfaces, our cookware, our crops and our earth, the widespread use of petrochemicals, the overuse of sunscreen, and now our electronic addictions. Each of these industries continues to commit untold crimes against our health, the health of our children and the health of our planet. The vaccine industry, however, leads the pack. Injecting foreign bodies, preservatives, animal cells, human embryo cells, pathogens and known carcinogenic adjuvants directly into the tissue (and bloodstream) of newly born infants and small children is the most vile and outrageous of all crimes. The assault on the undeveloped immune system cannot be understated.

If you suspect your child to have been damaged by vaccines, there are dietary, supplementary and chelation protocols you can follow for recovery. Used alongside homeopathy, reversal of Autoxic symptoms is possible. The earlier you start to detox your child, the better.

A Word About Families ~

Families are often our most important support groups. Even when we don't necessarily agree or get on, they are our pack. If you have decided on a more natural path but it interferes with your relationships, find a way. In conflict resolution, there is always a third way. You can remain firm in your convictions without upsetting your support system. I have many friends and very close family members who are as pro-medicine, science and vaccines as I am pro natural healing, earth wisdom and natural immunity. Over the years, we have come to an understanding that neither of us will change our opinions any time soon, but we refuse to let that separate us or come between the deep love and respect we have for one another. We have found a third way. There is room in our hearts for these great differences.

UNPACKING VACCINES

The vaccine issue is complicated and far beyond the scope of this book. It can be broken down into five main areas, each a minefield on its own. Scratch the surface of any of them and you will be led to obvious truths which have been purposefully hidden by the slickest and sickest of all industries- the marketing arms of the leading pharmaceutical vaccine manufacturers- Pfizer[10], Merk and Co[11]., GlaxoSmithKline[12], Johnson and Johnson[13] to name a few. Each guilty as charged, for knowingly misleading the public, so why would you trust them with your family's health? They have an openly stated fiscal (financial) responsibility and allegiance to their shareholders, not to you or your child or your family. They worship at the altar of greed and corruption, sacrificing our children to their gods and they will stop at nothing to make a profit.

Some areas to research:

1. Corruption and Conflicts of Interest in the Pharmaceutical Industry.

The conflicts of interests in the vaccine and pharmaceutical industries should shock anyone with an ounce of morality in their bones to the core. It is more than deeply disturbing that after overseeing the development of a vaccine, heads of pharmaceutical companies leave their positions only to become board members or CEOs of government bodies such as the CDC or WHO who influence decisions on vaccine requirements. A simple search on ECOSIA (not Google) will bring up any number of articles illustrating the depth of corruption.

Plague of Corruption - Restoring Faith in the Promise of Science, written by Judy Mikovits PhD, is well worth reading as is her first book, *Plague*.

Further research:

- Influence over media
- Influence over research outcomes
- Influence over medical journals
- Incentives to medical centers, hospitals and doctors

2. Inaccuracies and underreporting of the VAERS System

---

[10] https://www.corp-research.org/pfizer

[11] https://www.drugwatch.com/manufacturers/merck/

[12] https://www.justice.gov/opa/pr/glaxosmithkline-plead-guilty-and-pay-3-billion-resolve-fraud-allegations-and-failure-report

[13] https://www.consumersafety.org/news/johnson-and-johnson-lawsuits/

A study of the Vaccine Adverse Events Reporting System (VAERS), conducted by Harvard Medical School states, "Adverse events from drugs and vaccines are common, but underreported. [...] Likewise, **fewer than 1% of vaccine adverse events are reported.** Low reporting rates preclude or slow the identification of 'problem' drugs and vaccines that endanger public health. New surveillance methods for drug and vaccine adverse effects are needed."

Following the study, an upgrade was recommended to the VAERS system, but, "Unfortunately, there was never an opportunity to perform system performance assessments because the necessary CDC contacts were no longer available and the CDC consultants responsible for receiving data were no longer responsive to our **multiple requests** to proceed with testing and evaluation." It begs the question, what happened to them?

3. National Childhood Vaccine Injury Act
Protecting pharmaceutical companies from litigation is one of the most discriminatory acts passed by a US government. Parents struggling with the shock and the costs of a vaccine injured child have no support or recourse of action against the drug companies who are a protected industry when it comes to vaccines. Instead, they are required to sue the government, at their own expense, in the only 'vaccine court' in the country, going up against the DA. Can you imagine?
Further research-

- Lack of fair legal representation for vaccine damaged children- the cost of suing through vaccine courts.
- Personal cost to families of vaccine damaged children
- Limitation of access to Vaccine Court

4. Vaccine Ingredients and Safety
Most of us believe our government agencies would never allow anything unsafe into the market. That is the role of food and drug agencies, surely? But did you know that Vaccines were originally designed as weapon of war, and because of this, they were categorized 'biologics' instead of pharmaceutical in order to be fast tracked. This has allowed

pharmaceutical companies to get around strict FDA procedures, and allowed vaccines to be introduced into the market with very little follow up time. For example, Hepatitis B vaccines were licensed to give to one day old babies in the US following trials which monitored adverse reactions for only four and five days.[14]

"Biological products include a wide range of products such as vaccines, blood and blood components, allergenics, somatic cells, gene therapy, tissues, and recombinant therapeutic proteins. Biologics can be composed of sugars, proteins, or nucleic acids or complex combinations of these substances, or may be living entities such as cells and tissues. Biologics are isolated from a variety of natural sources- human, animal, or microorganism - and may be produced by biotechnology methods and other cutting-edge technologies"- FDA definition.

I implore all parents to demand and read the insert of any drug they use or give their children, so they are well aware of the effects and dangers as well as the ingredients. Vaccines by their very nature are designed to create an immune response. For this some toxic agents must be used. In the past that toxic agent was mercury in the MMR vaccine, and today it is still used as adjuvant in the flu shot given to pregnant women. The DTap, or TDaP uses aluminum as an adjuvant. See Professor Chris Exley on the effects of Aluminum in the brain. The Vaccine Guide by Ashley Everly can be downloaded from her website https://vaccine.guide

5. Vaccine Efficacy
- Differentiating between first and third world countries
- Timeline of decline in disease before mass vaccinations
- The cost to our health- vaccinated vs unvaccinated studies

It is rare to find a true double-blind placebo study. Control groups in almost all studies use children who have already been vaccinated. The claim being, that it would be unethical to

---

[14] For example, there are two Hepatitis B vaccines licensed for one day old babies in the United States – one manufactured by Merck and the other by GlaxoSmithKline. Merck's Hepatitis B vaccine was licensed by the FDA after trials which solicited adverse reactions for *only five days* after vaccination. Similarly, GlaxoSmithKline's Hepatitis B vaccine was licensed by the FDA after trials which solicited adverse reactions for *only four days* after vaccination. Introduction to Vaccine Safety Science & Policy in the United States - www.icandecide.org

deny a child a vaccine for the sake of the study. This is the kind of nonsense we consistently hear from the vaccine industry.

Like medical journalist Dell Bigtree says, it's like testing for the effects of alcohol by giving everyone a glass of whiskey and then giving half the group a beer chaser. This is how most of the testing is done. Group A get a vaccine with an aluminum adjuvant, and nothing else, and group B gets a vaccine with an aluminum adjuvant and a pathogen. The aluminum adjuvant is what causes the inflammatory response.

If these studies were done using honest placebo control groups (meaning one groups gets a saline vaccine, the other a regular vaccine), the results would generate such a loss of confidence in the vaccine and medical industries that it would open a pandoras box.

As we have witnessed over the past twenty years, any professional that dares to challenge the status quo is immediately subjected to the worst and most slanderous pharma-sponsored media trial. These include the esteemed and heroic Andrew Wakefield and Judy Mikovits to name a few. But the list grows daily as medical practitioners witness first-hand, the manipulative and controlling arms of pharma in their practices and as social media censorship becomes their new tool for control. The covid-19 narrative, has been a grand wake up call to physicians with a sense of justice and integrity and again many have lost or stand to lose their careers for challenging the all-powerful pharma subsidized health industries.

I believe vaccine damage is the cause of many physical, emotional, and mental health issues which plague our children today. I see it in my practice. The majority of children I treat who have not been vaccinated respond quickly to the correct remedy. The ones who have been vaccinated tend to be much more complicated to treat and often do not respond as expected, if ever, until they are detoxified (as much as possible), and even that has limitations and must be started as early as possible.

If you want to make your life and the life of your child easier, don't vaccinate them. I do not believe we have the right to inject something into a child's body without their consent, unless they are in a critical or life-threatening state. Vaccinations are not preventative; vitamin C and sunshine is preventative.

●●●

CHAPTER 9

My Cauldron

Let food be thy medicine, and medicine be thy food

Hippocrates

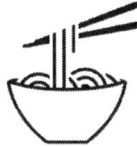

Recipes

After the birth of a child, in times of low energy, poor health or imbalance, through all the food wisdoms I have added to my cauldron over the years, I always return to the simple dishes I learned to prepare during those early macro days. Miso soup with a strip of mineral rich kombu seaweed, slow baked sweet root veg. or a simple pot of rice with steamed greens. When new moms in my community give birth, I like to make them a pot of Gia Jow- mothers brew, a traditional Chinese Chicken soup, which I adapted from a small macrobiotic book I bought when I first started on my journey as a new mom, called *Mother Love*.

Basic Stock

It's actually very easy to throw together a simple stock. Whenever you cook anything with vegetables, throw all the peels, roots and shavings into a pot of water. Add a strip of Kombu seaweed, and simmer on very low for a few hours. Strain and refrigerate or freeze the liquid.

You can transform your basic stock into a delicious Dashi broth by adding Bonita flakes (available at health food and Asian stores). Now, you have a very simple and delicious Asian soup broth base. Into this you can drop some thinly sliced carrots, pre-soaked shiitake mushrooms and thinly sliced onion. Cook till the vegetables are soft and then add cooked Asian noodles. (You can also add slices of steamed chicken, thinly sliced raw grass-fed beef which will cook in the heat of the soup, strips of egg omelet, tofu, whatever you like.) Season with a little good quality soy-sauce. If you like miso soup, stir in a few TBS Miso paste (to taste). Be sure NOT to bring to a boil once you have added the miso, as miso is a live culture and you don't want to kill off any living organisms. Top with toasted sesame seeds and shallots.

Traditional Jewish Chicken Soup

To a large pot add 1 small whole organic chicken and 1 kg of chicken wings. (You can just use wings which I do often, or you can add the neck of a turkey and some chicken frames or turkey bones). Add 1 large white onion, 4-6 peeled carrots, 1 whole sweet, red capsicum (Bell pepper), 2-4 sticks of celery, and a nice chunk of pumpkin. (You can also add celeriac or any seasonal soup vegetables). Cover with water or Basic Stock and bring to simmer. Clean off any scum that rises to the top and turn down the flame to a very low simmer. After 2-3 hours, add 5-6 cloves of fresh garlic, a slice of fresh ginger, some finely grated fresh turmeric, and half a bunch of fresh parsley. Add 1/2 Tbsp sweet paprika, and 1/2 Tbsp smoked paprika, 1Tbsp ground turmeric, salt and pepper to taste. Continue cooking on low for 4-6 hours. Add the rest of the parsley in the last ten minutes of cooking.

I sometimes serve this soup as it is, and sometimes I add a natural chicken stock or instead of the basic stock, I use a beef bone stock to change it up a bit.

Gluten free Dumplings

A story of gluten free dumplings...

When my son was five, he started to show signs of behavioral issues at school. The principle suggested he might be Autistic. I corrected her saying he's Artistic, not Autistic, but actually what he was, was Autoxic. I agreed to have an assessment providing she give me some time to detox him from whatever it was that was affecting his behavior. It was during this gluten-free period in our home that I adjusted Blue Greenberg's traditional Jewish matzah dumpling recipe into this delicious gluten-free version.

Even though the principle's diagnosis was wrong, I discovered an online community of guilt-ridden parents desperately trying to detox their vaccine damaged children. I followed their protocols, doing cartwheels in the kitchen and after two years of healing his damaged gut, my son was able to return to a normal diet and lifestyle, with the addition of a few supplements. He was neither Oppositional, nor Autistic, he was, as I had suspected, Autoxic,- a word I have used ever since to describe our vaccine and environmentally damaged children.

In many ways my fight for the cause has remained steadfast throughout the years in support of the courageous parents who shared their stories and information so generously with me. Jan Brenton, was one of the pioneers of the movement in Australia. I reference her book entitled, *Can we manage Autism, Yes we Can,* often in my practice. It is a wonderful reference for any parent trying to detoxify their child.

RECIPE

Break up 12 rice crackers. Add 1/4 cup of hot cooked chicken soup, 1 tsp salt, ground black pepper and 4 eggs. The hot soup will soften the rice crackers. Use

a potato masher to further break up the crackers till all the ingredients form a firm but damp mix. Refrigerate for at least 3 hours. Form into balls and

drop into boiling seasoned water/stock or soup. Cook for a few minutes, till the balls turn themselves over and look light and fluffy. These are ridiculously delicious in traditional chicken soup.

Gai Jow - Mother's Brew

This is the most wonderfully nourishing meal for new mothers.

Soak 8 dry shitake mushrooms, 6-8 pieces of Chinese black wood fungus, a quarter of a cup raw peanuts and 20 Lilly buds (all available from Asian grocers) in separate bowls of water till soft. Cut off all the hard bits, tie a knot into each Lilly bud, and add all to Traditional Chicken soup for the last hour of cooking. (When I make this for new mothers, I make the above traditional chicken soup recipe with less spices, making the soup very mild)

Just before you remove the soup from the heat, add 1/4 glass of whiskey, cook off the alcohol and serve.

Seasonal Steamed Greens

There is little I love more than to pick an assortment of greens from my garden, rinse them off and throw them into a salad or steam them.

Wash a bunch of mixed greens- Bok Choy, spinach, kale, Chinese greens, baby broccoli, snow peas, mustard greens, string beans, whatever is local, seasonal and fresh. Heat up a pan and add a dash of Olive oil. Throw in the greens and stir for a few minutes. They should retain their wonderful rich green color and still be a little crunchy to eat. Add a splash of soy sauce and a good squeeze of lemon juice. Serve over a bed of basmati rice, or with Asian noodles or if you are avoiding grains, just eat as they are.

Simple Asian Garlic Noodles

I love this quick delicious meal. It was a staple when my kids were small because it's so easy to throw together. It can be served with a piece of grilled chicken or fish and steamed greens.

Heat up a pan, add a good few tablespoons of olive oil. Add cooked Udon noodles, though any Asian noodles will do. Stir adding a dash of good quality soy sauce and some freshly crushed garlic.

Baked Root Veg

In a baking dish, chop into large chunks: 1 medium Jap pumpkin (or any sweet pumpkin), 3-4 beets, 3 sweet potatoes and a medium white onion. Add 3-4 Tbsp of olive oil 2 Tbsp of Mirin- Japanese cooking wine, and 2 Tbsp soy sauce (or to taste). Sprinkle with fresh Rosemary and cover with baking paper and seal with (recycled) aluminum foil. Bake in a moderate oven for 40 minutes and then uncover and grill or continue roasting for another 10 minutes or till the vegetables crisp up a bit.

Sour-dough Starter Culture

Before supermarkets and refrigeration, we all made bread at home. It's much easier than you think. The internet is full of wonderful videos and websites. A favorite is Mike Greenfield who will show you how to turn this easy starter into a delicious home-made sour-dough bread with nothing more than flour, water and salt.

Here is the simplest way to make your own starter culture.

Make up a mix of good quality flour and water using 1 cup of flour: 1/2 cup water. Be sure to use good quality filtered or spring water, and a clean bowl. Cover with a soft cloth and let stand in a warm spot in your kitchen until it starts to show live activity. Bubbles will start to gather on the surface, and it will start to smell earthy.

This is a live culture, so it needs to be fed. Once the starter is alive with yeast it has picked up from your kitchen, you will need to feed it daily. To get a good active culture you need to feed it almost as much in volume as the mix itself by adding a few tablespoons of flour daily. So, as it grows in size, you will have to throw out some of your culture to be able to continue feeding it without going through too much flour (food).

Mike Greenfield suggests frying up a delicious salted, savory pancake with what you throw off each day, which I often do, to the delight of my hungry teenage kids. You can find his recipe on YouTube in his clip entitled, 15 Mistakes Most Beginner Sourdough Bakers Make.

Fermented Cabbage ~ Sauerkraut

Slice or shred 1 whole head of white cabbage. Add 1 Tbsp good quality kosher or raw sea salt and scrunch it up with your hands for about 3 minutes until the cabbage softens a little and starts to release its own juice. Leave to stand for 10 minutes. Stuff into a clean glass mason jar, pushing the cabbage down with your fist until it is covered by its own liquid. Cover the top with some of the washed outside leaves and make sure you leave a good 5 cm or more between the top of the liquid and the lid. Keep the top submerged using the root of the cabbage. Close and leave to sit in a warm spot in your kitchen for 4-7 days depending on the temperature.

You will see the fermentation take place. The liquid will start to bubble and come alive. Store in a cool place for 1-4 weeks and refrigerate when it tastes a little fermented, and vinegary, like sauerkraut. Store in the fridge and eat some every day to encourage good gut bacteria. If this is a new food, introduce it slowly. Best served with meat, though beneficial any time.

You can add carrots, beets, purple cabbage, ginger, garlic, chili or whatever you like to your fermented vegetables. Experiment and have fun.

Medicine Pantry

I recommend parents invest in a small first aid kid from the pharmacy, which includes some light bandages, clean glaze, sterile wipes, and some antiseptic solution and some strike tape for emergencies. Here is a list of natural products to keep in your medicine pantry.

Hydrogen Peroxide antiseptic, to keep newly pierced ears clean or to clean open wounds. Be sure to use according to instructions. **High alcohol solution** will do the same thing.
Coconut oil is an anti-bacterial. You can use it to swish around your mouth and through your teeth every morning for a few minutes (called pulling) to keep your mouth clean. It is also good for gut health and is a superb fat for underweight children or teens. It can be applied topically on wounds and mild skin irritations. It can be used as an anti-fungal, a natural deodorant and a natural lip balm.
Saline solution for sore or tired eyes and washing over wounds to clean them.
Saline nasal spray for congestion. Be sure not to share from one family member to the next.

Sodium bicarbonate (baking soda) neutralizes acid. If you suffer from excess acidity, you can add 1/4 tsp sodium bicarbonate to a glass of water and drink it first thing every morning. I also suggest giving this to children when they have eaten bad foods or are feeling unwell.

Lavender oil increases circulation and relaxes the nervous system. It can be added to a warm bath or to an oil diffuser or burner to settle overactive children or over exhausted parents. It can be used to treat ringworm and rubbed on the temples to relieve a headache.

Tea-tree oil- antiseptic, anti-fungal, anti-bacterial.

Salt can be mixed into cold or iced water to treat minor household skin burns. Used as a mouth gargle, an antiseptic, to relax tired muscles. To balance excessive sugar intake.

Epsom Salt in a bath can counter the effects of too much chlorine in a pool. It helps increase glutathione which helps with detoxification. The magnesium compound helps relax muscles.

Calendula salve is excellent for burns, wounds, eczema, bites, skin rashes and allergic skin reactions.

> **Calendula Salve Recipe:** Add 1 cup of fresh calendula flowers to enough olive oil to just cover. Store away from direct light for 6 weeks. Strain. On a very low flame, warm up grated beeswax. Add it to the infused oil. You will need 1TBS of beeswax: 30ml oil. You can add other healing herbs such as Lavender, Hypericum and Comfrey.[15]

Olive leaf extract is a strong anti-viral.

Manuka Honey is an excellent antibacterial.

Zinc oxide makes an excellent non-toxic sun block and provides the body with zinc.

Aloe Vera can be used to treat sunburn and as a topical cream to relieve burning.

Echinacea stimulates the immune system.

Elderberry is an antioxidant, high in Vitamin C.

Vitamin C- can take the edge off any infection. I advise parents to use it generously when their children are coming down with a cold or flu, or have a bite, cut or any type of infection. See Suzanne Humphrey protocols.

---

[15] Thanks to Medicine woman and Herbalist Orli Lauffer for this recipe from her course in Wild Foraging in Israel

Vitamin D- during winter or if you live in a sun starved part of the world.

Zinc - most of us are deficient as is our soil. You can buy liquid zinc and do the taste test to check if you are deficient.

Vitamin A is essential for the treatment of measles and sunburn.

Vaccine Education Resources

You can use the search engine ECOSIA, which will deliver less biased results than Google, who have pharmaceutical interests. If you would like to understand more, here are some reputable sites and references. This list is far from extensive, rather it is an opening for anyone that wishes to do more research.

The National Vaccine Information Centre- https://www.nvic.org

The Children's Health Defense- Robert Kennedy Jr. - https://childrenshealthdefense.org

I Can Decide- Dell Bigtree- https://www.icandecide.org

The High Wire- Dell Bigtree

Andrew Wakefield

      Vaxxed- From Cover Up to Catastrophe

      Andrew Wakefield- The Pathological Optimist,

      Dr. Andrew Wakefield Deals with Allegations.

Also, worth reading: The Real Story of Dr. Andrew Wakefield and MMR (by Mary Holland, JD)

The Untrivial Pursuit- Joy M Fritz (also on telegram)

The Vaccine Guide- Ashley Everly – Toxologist, https://vaccine.guide

Professor Chris Exley- Aluminium in Human Brain Tissue

Dr Tetyana Obukhanych, Ph.D.- Natural Immunity and Vaccination

Doctors to follow:

Dr. Suzanne Humphries- Nephrologist, see her Vitamin C protocols and treatments for Whooping cough and Tetanus.

Dr. Larry Polevsky- Pediatrician, see what he has to say about fevers.

Dr. Peter Gotzsche- Deadly Medicines and Organised Crime- How Big Pharma Has Corrupted Health Care.

Dr. Peter Gotzsche- Exposing Big Pharma as Organised Crime

Medical Journals Are an Extension of the Marketing Arm of Pharmaceutical Companies- Pubmed

Books and References

Organon of Medicine, Samuel Hahnemann

The Homeopathic Materia Medicas and Repertories of:

Boericke, Kent, Allan, Nash, Dunham, Farrington and Vithoulkas

The Science of Homeopathy, George Vithoulkas

Levels of Health (2nd volume 3rd revised edition), George Vithoulkas

Materia Medica Viva- Vithoulkas- The International Academy of Classical Homeopathy.

Essence of Materia Medica Second Edition, George Vithoulkas

The Homeopathic Treatment of Children, Paul Herscu N.D.

Homeopathy, A Home Prescriber, Phyllis Speight

Your Healthy Child with Homeopathy, Tricia Allans

Nourishing Traditions, Sally Fallon

How to Talk So Kids Will Listen and Listen So Kids Will Talk, Adele Faber, Elaine Mazlish

Women Who Run with the Wolves, Clarissa Pinkola Estes

Can we manage Autism, Yes we Can, Jan Brenton

Plague of Corruption - Restoring Faith in the Promise of Science, Judy Mikovits PhD,

Dr. Zach Bush- https://zachbushmd.com

Mike Greenfield- YouTube.

Printed in Great Britain
by Amazon